Mindfulness-Oriented Recovery Enhancement

Mindfulness-Oriented Recovery Enhancement

An Evidence-Based Treatment for Chronic Pain and Opioid Use

Eric L. Garland

THE GUILFORD PRESS
New York   London

The author has checked with sources believed to be reliable in his efforts to provide information
that is complete and generally in accord with the standards of practice that are accepted at the
time of publication. However, in view of the possibility of human error or changes in behavioral,
mental health, or medical sciences, neither the author, nor the editor and publisher, nor any other
party who has been involved in the preparation or publication of this work warrants that the
information contained herein is in every respect accurate or complete, and they are not responsible
for any errors or omissions or the results obtained from the use of such information. Readers are
encouraged to confirm the information contained in this book with other sources.

Library of Congress Cataloging-in-Publication Data

Names: Garland, Eric L., author.
Title: Mindfulness-oriented recovery enhancement : an evidence-based treatment for chronic pain
    and opioid use / Eric L Garland.
Description: New York : The Guilford Press, [2024] | Includes bibliographical references and index.
Identifiers: LCCN 2024014596 | ISBN 9781462554867 (trade paperback ; alk. paper) |
    ISBN 9781462554874 (hardcover ; alk. paper)
Subjects: MESH: Opioid-Related Disorders—therapy | Pain Management | Mindfulness |
    BISAC: PSYCHOLOGY / Psychopathology / Addiction | MEDICAL / Nursing / Psychiatric &
    Mental Health
Classification: LCC RC568.O45 | NLM WM 284 | DDC 615.7/822—dc23/eng/20240424
LC record available at *https://lccn.loc.gov/2024014596*

To my parents, wife, and children: Your love has nourished me, sustained me, and helped me to reach this moment to share this work with the world.

To the great teachers (intellectual and spiritual) whose wisdom pervades this work and links it in an unbroken chain to the Source.

Finally, to the many patients with whom I have had the honor to work over the decades: Thank you for teaching me to walk the path of healing.

About the Author

Eric L. Garland, PhD, LCSW, is Distinguished Endowed Chair in Research, Distinguished Professor, and Associate Dean for Research at the University of Utah College of Social Work, where he is also Director of the Center on Mindfulness and Integrative Health Intervention Development. Dr. Garland is the developer of Mindfulness-Oriented Recovery Enhancement. He has published more than 250 scientific papers and has conducted extensive clinical trials of mindfulness for addiction and chronic pain. Dr. Garland is an appointed member of the Multi-Disciplinary Working Group that assists the Helping to End Addiction Long-term Initiative of the National Institutes of Health (NIH HEAL Initiative). In 2021, a bibliometric analysis of mindfulness research published over the past 55 years found Dr. Garland to be the most prolific author of mindfulness research in the world.

Preface

Life is a precious gift. The very breath that fills our lungs is given to us each moment. Yet life is also beset by suffering. Our embodiment, though it offers nearly endless opportunities to experience blissful pleasure, is also capable of feeling great pain. Such is the human condition: We get sick, we get old, and we die. And we resist and rail against the perceived injustice of our fate. In so doing, we unwittingly magnify our own pain. We bring anguish upon ourselves by trying to avoid pain and hardship.

To avoid suffering, many people have turned to mind-altering drugs. This route has been taken for millennia. For instance, the ancient Greeks used opium to relieve emotional as well as physical pain (Dormandy, 2012). In *The Odyssey*, Homer described such use:

> Into the bowl in which their wine was mixed, she slipped a drug that had the power of robbing grief and anger of their sting and banishing all painful memories. No one who swallowed this dissolved in their wine could shed a single tear that day, even for the death of his mother or father. (ca. 700 B.C.E./1946, p. 70)

Given the ability of opioids to numb the soul to pain and loss, it is no wonder that we have turned to these powerful drugs not just for relief from physical pain but also in search of an emotional respite—an escape from the anxieties, injustice, isolation, and other forms of suffering that exist in the communities where we live. In the modern era, savvy marketers have promised such an escape through appealing messages exhorting us to enjoy the benefits of ever-more powerful, synthetic versions of the drug Homer sang about so long ago.

This appeal was real—opioids can, in fact, provide temporary relief from physical pain and despair. When the gnawing ache of chronic pain is quelled, when one's spirits are lifted after months or years of depression and anxiety, one may feel something akin to bliss. But the true bliss of happiness it is not. In fact, the sensation produced is more often dullness and a loss of feeling, not the presence of joy. Yet, as a means of momentary respite from overwhelming, immobilizing pain, prescribing these drugs could been seen as humane and an act of compassion. Unfortunately, their very potency too easily blinds us to their malign effects. Who should deny the uplifting possibility of being pain-free and functional after months or years of unrelenting torment? Ironically, due to the very ways in which chronic opioid use changes the function of the human nervous system, this promise of relief often goes unfulfilled. Gradually, and insidiously, the pain-relieving effects of these drugs weaken over time as we suffer from the pangs of withdrawal in their absence, even as we come to see opioids as more and more necessary to our ability to function. As a consequence of this process, some people are compelled to take higher and higher doses of the drug just to feel okay, which paradoxically causes them to feel more anguish and fall into a downward spiral of increasing dependence that prevents one from finding anything like a solution to the problem of chronic pain.

This book presents one part of the solution. Although there are a number of helpful treatments for chronic pain and substance use, in our fragmented health care system, these conditions are typically addressed separately. Such a disjointed approach is doomed from the start, insofar as the downward spiral linking chronic pain to opioid misuse and opioid use disorder (OUD) involves feedback loops that perpetuate and exacerbate this comorbidity. Distinct from typical treatments that treat chronic pain and opioid use separately, this book describes an innovative, integrative, and evidence-based therapeutic approach: Mindfulness-Oriented Recovery Enhancement (MORE). MORE was designed to simultaneously address chronic pain, emotional distress, and substance use. We know that co-occurring disorders are very common: About 50% of individuals with an OUD (or other substance use disorder) also have chronic pain (Delorme et al., 2023; John & Wu, 2020), and approximately one-third have a psychiatric disorder like major depression or anxiety (Santo et al., 2022). Similarly, about one-quarter of people with chronic pain misuse opioids (Vowles et al., 2015), and mental health problems are strongly associated with opioid misuse (Rogers et al., 2021). MORE provides a core set of therapeutic skills that can be used to help heal these complex comorbidities. MORE also stands out from other addiction treatments in that it provides training in unique, mind–body techniques that aim to increase the sense of natural healthy pleasure, joy, meaning, and self-transcendence—teaching people in recovery how to use their minds to access an inner wellspring of well-being to make themselves feel good, naturally.

This description of MORE's therapeutic focus is not a mere platitude but actually speaks to its core mechanisms of action, for the very neural substrates of chronic pain and opioid addiction involve a dysregulation of the brain's reward system. As alluded to earlier, when trapped in the downward spiral, the individual becomes dulled to life's pleasures and empty inside, seeking an external means to fill this void, and becomes increasingly dependent upon a drug that insidiously robs one from feeling a sense of contentment outside of the fleeting satisfaction that comes from perpetually feeding an insatiable hunger. Unlike many of the extant psychological treatments for chronic pain and addictive behavior that were developed well before the advent of modern neuroscience, MORE emerged at a time when science began to develop a clearer understanding of how substance use and psychiatric disorders, as well as chronic pain conditions, disrupt the structure and function of brain circuits undergirding cognitive and affective processes integral to human flourishing. MORE was developed with these neuroscientific discoveries in mind, and thus this therapy represents a significant advance for the fields of behavioral health, chronic pain treatment, and addiction medicine. Yet, at the same time, MORE is rooted in age-old contemplative philosophy and practices intended to extinguish attachment to the sense of an isolated and skin-encapsulated ego. Although many philosophical and spiritual systems have long held that clinging to the sense of an independent, isolated self is the root of suffering, it is only in the past several decades that neuroscientific research has revealed an association between our default mode habits of ruminative self-referential processing and a range of psychiatric maladies. MORE aims to help people transcend these limiting self-views and taste one's true nature as part of an interconnected oneness with something greater than the self-in-isolation. Thus, the MORE therapeutic approach represents a true integration of ancient wisdom and modern science.

MORE unites three great traditions within psychotherapy—mindfulness training, cognitive-behavioral therapy (CBT), and positive psychology—into a manualized, evidence-based treatment, developed and tested over the course of 15 years of scientific research and clinical practice. The first version of the MORE treatment manual was published nearly a decade ago in a seminal and critically important text for clinicians who work with people suffering from a wide array of substance use disorders (Garland, 2013). In the years that followed, the MORE model was significantly modified and updated to address the specific and complex comorbidity of chronic pain, opioid misuse, and OUD among people prescribed long-term opioid analgesic therapy. Although the original MORE manual presented some initial and preliminary guidance pertaining to these complicated clinical targets in a protean form, the book you hold in your hands today represents the fully developed, fully refined, and state-of-the-art approach to using MORE to address chronic pain and opioid use, an approach that has been vetted in multiple randomized clinical trials. Furthermore, this text clearly outlines the complex, interlocking, neuropsychopharmacological mechanisms that propel the downward spiral from chronic pain to opioid use and addiction. Armed with this conceptual understanding, you will be well equipped to implement MORE for this specific population of patients for whom few evidence-based treatment options are available.

This book uses nongendered pronouns to align with modern style and convention, and throughout the text, I refer to the concepts of *opioid misuse* and *opioid addiction*. These terms are not meant to be pejorative but rather descriptive of the clinical phenomena under question. Opioid misuse refers to the use of opioids in ways other than prescribed. For example, many people take higher opioid doses than prescribed and, consequently, run out of medication prior to their next refill. Sometimes, facing a shortage of medication, people seek opioids from multiple prescribers, or obtain illicit opioids from the street (e.g., heroin, fentanyl). It is also not uncommon to use opioids to allay emotional distress, produce euphoria, or to facilitate sleep, none of which are indications approved by the U.S. Food and Drug Administration (FDA) for this type of medication. These behaviors alone do not indicate the presence of opioid addiction (or OUD), but often presage the development of addiction. Opioid addiction constitutes a progressive loss of control over opioid use that typically involves compulsive behavior and serious social or health consequences. To be clear, not all people with chronic pain who are prescribed opioid analgesic medications misuse them or become addicted to them. In fact, most don't. MORE can also be helpful for individuals with chronic pain who have not progressed to opioid misuse or addiction, insofar as the MORE therapeutic approach can produce powerful pain relief, reduce stress, and strengthen self-awareness. This book describes in detail how to use MORE to help a diverse array of patients alleviate physical and emotional pain, reduce opioid use, prevent opioid misuse, and recover from opioid addiction. Over the years since MORE's inception, therapists have implemented the model with thousands of such patients to great effect, and this book represents a distillation of the practice wisdom derived from those efforts.

Acknowledgments

Given that "no man is an island," I would like to acknowledge and offer a deep bow of gratitude to the many mentors, colleagues, and loved ones without whom this work would never have seen the light of day:

My beloved father and mother, Howard and Eileen Garland, who gave me the gifts of awareness, inquiry, and savoring, all of which are entwined into the heart of MORE.

My PhD mentors Matthew Howard, Susan Gaylord, and Barbara Fredrickson, who believed in me and taught the basic skills and theoretical frameworks that informed the MORE research program.

My graduate school professor Mark Fraser, who prompted the development of the first version of the MORE manual.

His Holiness the Dalai Lama and the Mind and Life Institute, who funded the initial research on MORE and who inspired my work to integrate contemplative science into a compassionate approach to alleviating human suffering.

My colleague Brett Froeliger, who helped me elucidate MORE through the lens of addiction neurobiology and who partnered with me to develop the restructuring reward hypothesis.

My many other colleagues with whom I have shared the "life of the mind" and who have helped advance the science underlying MORE and its implementation, including Nina Cooperman, John Barrett, Rita Goldstein, Chantal Martin-Soelch, Fadel Zeidan, David Vago, Patrick Finan, Yoshi Nakamura, Justin Hudak, Norman Farb, Ben Lewis, Philippe Goldin, Siri Leknes, Aleksandra Zgierska, Rob Edwards, Dan Rhon, Julie Fritz, Linda Carlson, Sahib Khalsa, Jun Mao, Chantal Berna, Spencer Dorn, Neil Abell, Tina Liu-Tom, and Nancy Sudak, among many others.

The National Institutes of Health and the U.S. Department of Defense, which have stalwartly supported the MORE research program for more than a decade.

Amber Kelly, Anne Baker, Anna Parisi, Kelly Hendrickson, and the many other talented therapists and graduate students from whom I learned as they delivered MORE to patients in multiple randomized clinical trials across the country.

Gary Donaldson, whose statistical wizardry revealed the effects of MORE in elegant mathematical equations.

My former mentee and now colleague Adam Hanley, whose creativity helped to expand the MORE program into innovative directions.

Jon Kabat-Zinn, a true inspiration and pioneer of modern mindfulness-based interventions, who grounded me in the strength of the dharma when I faltered.

The many sages and gurus of Kashmir Shaivism, Taoism, Mahāmudrā, Dzogchen, and Kabbalah whose ideas implicitly and explicitly flow through this work in a lineage extending through history, straight from the Source.

My dear friends (you know who you are), who have danced with me through my self-transcendent moments and have given me so many opportunities to savor life.

My auntie Linda and mother-in-law, Peggy, who kvelled for me when my parents couldn't.

My brother, Adam, whose wise counsel and caring presence has been a blessing.

My children, Ari and Eden, who help me remember what really matters in life and who represent my hope for the future.

And, finally, my wife, Lisa, the love of my life, without whom this work would not have been possible. Lisa, you are my rock and my foundation.

So, with the support of many beautiful hearts and minds, I give you this book—the culmination of many years of science and therapy that have touched the lives of so many people in need. May our collective work, as agents of unity and compassion, help to heal suffering and advance human flourishing.

Preface

My dear friends (you know who you are), who have danced with me through my self-transcendent moments and have given me so many opportunities to savor life.

My aunt, Linda and mother-in-law, Peggy who kvelled for me when my parents could be.

My brother, Adam, whose wise counsel and caring presence has been a blessing.

My children, Ari and Eden, who help me remember what really matters in life and who represent my hope for the future.

And, finally, my wife, Lisa, the love of my life, without whom this work would not have been possible. Lisa, you are my rock and my foundation.

So with the support of many beautiful hearts and minds, I give you this book—the culmination of many years of science and therapy that have touched the lives of so many people in need. May our collective work, as agents of unity and compassion, help to heal suffering and advance human flourishing.

Contents

The MORE Sessions

Chapter 1

Introduction

In 2015, Nobel Prize-winning economists Anne Case and Angus Deaton found that for the first time in many decades, the mortality rate among U.S. middle-aged adults was rising precipitously, which they attributed in large part to the opioid crisis (Case & Deaton, 2015)—a crisis that has been termed a "disease of despair" in the epidemiological and sociological literatures (Stein et al., 2017). This term is not a mere metaphor but actually strikes right at the heart of the pathogenic mechanisms driving this crisis. For indeed, despair has fueled the opioid crisis into a conflagration, a raging fire that has consumed countless lives all the way through today.

The disease of despair has many sources, from the rising tide of income inequality to the lack of opportunity, from intergenerational violence and trauma to the egocentric materialism and social isolation of modern culture—so empty of the humanistic values that once guided and anchored our ancestors in a collective bond. In the face of this vacuum of meaning, it was perhaps inevitable that life would become more painful, insofar as emotional pain begets physical pain in the brain (Wiech & Tracey, 2009). Indeed, rates of chronic pain have soared across all Western societies, but perhaps nowhere more severely than in the United States, where an estimated 50 million Americans experience chronic pain per year (Dahlhamer et al., 2018).

How the Opioid Crisis Began

The opioid crisis arose in part due to well-intentioned efforts to alleviate untreated pain. For much of the 20th century, opioids were prescribed primarily for postoperative and cancer-related pain. However, fueled by misleading and unethical marketing practices of certain pharmaceutical companies (Keefe, 2021), in the 1990s prescription of opioids to treat all forms of pain became part of the standard of care, and consequently, opioid prescriptions climbed to 208 million by 2011. By 2015, approximately 38% of the U.S. adult population had used prescription opioids in the prior 12 months (Han et al., 2017). Though opioids have been thought to be useful in managing a wide continuum of pain from acute and procedural pain to chronic pain, evidence for their long-term efficacy and safety is limited (Chou et al., 2015). Surprisingly, few studies have demonstrated whether the immediate, pain-relieving effects of opioids persist when opioids are taken over the years to address long-standing chronic pain. To the contrary, it is well-known that regular use of opioids leads to specific neuroadaptations resulting in *tolerance*, whereby an individual must take higher and higher opioid doses to achieve the same degree of pain relief. And prolonged, high-dose use of opioid analgesics can inadvertently lead to other hazards, including opioid overdose, opioid misuse, and the development of opioid use disorder (OUD). Indeed, the dramatic increase in opioid prescriptions in the first decade of the 21st century was accompanied by a rising incidence of opioid misuse and OUD that affected 8.5 million and 6.5 million Americans (respectively) in 2022 (Substance Abuse and Mental Health Services Administration [SAMHSA], 2023).

Misuse of prescription opioids continues to dwarf the heroin problem in the United States, with misuse of opioids like oxycodone, hydrocodone, and fentanyl being 17 times more prevalent than heroin use (SAMHSA, 2023). The opioid crisis only worsened under COVID-19 (Becker & Fiellin, 2020)—with a 38.4% increase in opioid deaths in May 2020 from the year before the declaration of the COVID-19 national emergency in the United States (Centers for Disease Control and Prevention, 2020). Though opioids are misused by people without pain, some individuals with chronic pain who are prescribed long-term opioid therapy (LTOT) are at heightened risk for opioid misuse and OUD. Meta-analytic estimates indicate that approximately 25.0% of people who are prescribed opioids for chronic pain engage in opioid misuse behaviors like taking higher doses than prescribed, obtaining opioids from multiple providers, or using opioids to alleviate symptoms other than pain (e.g., to relieve negative emotional states like sadness, anxiety, or anger; Vowles et al., 2015). Approximately 10.0% of people on LTOT go on to experience the loss of control over opioid use that distinguishes OUD from opioid misuse (Vowles et al., 2015).

Addressing opioid misuse and OUD is complex and difficult in its own right, but the comorbidity of chronic pain increases this difficulty significantly. Indeed, chronic pain worsens OUD treatment outcomes (Potter et al., 2010; Worley et al., 2015) and significantly increases risk of relapse for patients treated with medications for opioid use disorder (MOUD; Vest et al., 2020)—the gold standard medical treatment for OUD. Chapter 2 details the downward spiral of behavioral escalation linking chronic pain to opioid misuse and OUD, but in brief, the pharmacological effects of prolonged opioid use on the brain increase sensitivity to emotional distress and physical pain while decreasing sensitivity to the pleasure derived from natural rewards in the social environment (Garland, Froeliger, Zeidan, et al., 2013; Koob, 2020). These neurobiological changes undermine the ability to regulate emotions, leading to dysphoria. Opioid dose escalation ensues in an effort to preserve a dwindling sense of well-being, which only serves to perpetuate and hasten the downward spiral, ensnaring the individual in a vicious cycle that magnifies pain and fuels addiction.

> Prolonged opioid use changes the brain by increasing sensitivity to pain while decreasing sensitivity to pleasure.

That said, not all people with chronic pain misuse opioids or become addicted to them; in fact, most don't. Yet, due to changes in opioid prescribing practices following publication of the 2016 Centers for Disease Control and Prevention opioid guidelines (Dowell et al., 2016), many people who were experiencing satisfactory levels of pain relief and who functioned well from opioid treatment are now suffering due to being forcibly and rapidly tapered off of opioids. Opioid tapering without the proper support has now been linked with an increased risk of mental health crises, suicide, and overdose (Agnoli et al., 2021; Mackey et al., 2020). So clearly, the many millions of people prescribed opioids for chronic pain cannot be asked to stop their opioid use without an effective alternative pain management approach. Given the reluctance of many health systems to continue to prescribe opioids to patients, there is a huge need for approaches to support people with chronic pain who once depended on opioids for pain relief. This unmet need only complicates the current opioid crisis even further, by driving some people who previously took opioid analgesics as prescribed by their physicians to the street in search of illicit opioids, including fentanyl and heroin, as a means of alleviating their anguish.

Due to the complexity of the mechanisms linking chronic pain to opioid misuse and OUD, successful treatments for opioid misuse and OUD among people with chronic pain have proven elusive. A 2015 National Institutes of Health–Agency for Healthcare Research and Quality systematic review found no evidence for the effectiveness of any interventions for reducing opioid misuse or addiction among people receiving LTOT for chronic pain (Chou et al., 2015). More than 9 years later this gap remains.

I developed Mindfulness-Oriented Recovery Enhancement (MORE) to fill this gap. Specifically, MORE is a mind–body therapy approach informed by discoveries from cognitive psychology, affective science, and neurobiology, as well as by ancient contemplative wisdom traditions (e.g., Mahāmudrā, Dzogchen, Nondual Shaiva Tantra), and select Western philosophies that emphasize the primacy of consciousness in human experience (e.g., second-order cybernetics, stoicism, phenomenology). MORE unites complementary aspects of mindfulness training, third-wave cognitive-behavioral therapy (CBT), and principles from positive psychology into an integrative treatment for addictive behavior, emotional distress, and chronic pain. MORE is a sequenced treatment. It begins with a foundation of mindfulness training, which by virtue of its effects on strengthening the mind, synergizes later training in reappraisal and savoring, which ultimately may lead toward self-transcendence, the sense of being connected to something greater than the self (see Figure 1.1). These treatment components are designed to activate a series of cognitive, affective, and physiological mechanisms that are in turn intended to produce stepwise change in a range of clinical targets relevant to the treatment of chronic pain, opioid misuse, and OUD. Chapter 2 describes these treatment targets. Then, Chapter 3 discusses the conceptual framework underlying MORE, with the remaining chapters and structured session guides thereafter describing the MORE program in detail.

> MORE is an integrative treatment for addictive behavior, emotional distress, and chronic pain.

This book describes how MORE can be used to support people with chronic pain and opioid-related issues. MORE may be useful for several types of patients. First, MORE can be used to treat people with chronic pain who are misusing or at risk for misusing opioids. Second, MORE can be used to treat people with chronic pain who have progressed to OUD and who may (or may not) be receiving addictions treatment. Third, MORE can be used to help people in chronic pain who are being asked by their physicians to taper their opioid medication. Finally, MORE can be used to support people who are seeking chronic pain relief and/or are self-motivated to reduce their opioid use or come off of opioids entirely. The MORE program, as detailed here, has been used successfully with all four of these types of patients.

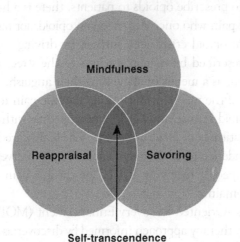

Mindfulness: Nonreactive attention to, and acceptance of, thoughts, emotions, and sensations, while cultivating awareness of the field of awareness itself (*meta-awareness*)

Reappraisal: Reframing the meaning of a stressful life event to see that event as benign, a source of growth, or a learning opportunity

Savoring: Focusing attention on the pleasant sensory features of an object or event, or its higher-order affective meaning, to increase the sense of reward obtained from the experience

Self-transcendence: Connecting to a source of meaning that is greater than the self

FIGURE 1.1. Visual representation of the MORE approach.

History of the MORE Program

In 2006, rooted in my own personal mindfulness practice and inspired by Jon Kabat-Zinn's (1982, 2003, 2011, 2019) seminal Mindfulness-Based Stress Reduction program and its later offshoot, Mindfulness-Based Cognitive Therapy (Segal et al., 2002, 2013; Teasdale et al., 2000), I began to contemplate developing a mindfulness-based intervention (MBI) for the treatment of addiction. At the time, there were no empirically supported mindfulness-based treatments for addiction, and few studies of mindfulness for addictive behavior had been published in the scientific literature. As one key exception, a quasi-experimental study of traditional vipassana meditation (Buddhist insight meditation) for incarcerated substance abusers had been published that year (Bowen et al., 2006). Motivated in part by this study, I saw the need for a secular mindfulness program for addiction that was founded on mechanistic insights from basic biobehavioral research and neuroscience. To begin, I first reviewed the literature on the cognitive, affective, and neurobiological mechanisms underpinning addiction. This review identified two key mechanistic targets that might be treated by mindfulness: *automaticity* and *allostasis*. With regard to the first mechanistic target, automaticity, research suggested that addiction was largely governed by unconscious cognitive and behavioral habits (Everitt & Robbins, 2016; Tiffany, 1990)—a conclusion echoed in the accounts of people with substance use disorders who described feeling automatically compelled to use substances even when they wished to abstain from drug use. As a manifestation of automaticity in addiction, people with substance use disorders exhibit an *attentional bias*, or hyperfixation of attention, toward cues associated with past drug use episodes (e.g., the sight of an opioid pill bottle), which can trigger craving for substances (Field & Cox, 2008). With regard to the second mechanistic target, allostasis, addiction neurobiology indicates that the progression to compulsive substance use involves an allostatic process (i.e., a process by which the body adapts and changes in response to stress in order to maintain internal equilibrium). Specifically, as mentioned earlier, prolonged drug use in the context of chronic stress increases sensitization to drug cues and aversive experiences (e.g., pain) while decreasing sensitivity to the healthy pleasure and meaning derived from natural rewards in the socioenvironment (e.g., food, sex, social relationships, the beauty of nature; Koob & Le Moal, 2001). This allostatic shift in brain stress and reward thresholds leads to an overwhelmingly negative emotional state, driving drug use as a means of self-medicating intense feelings of dysphoria and anxiety, and trapping the individual in a downward spiral of escalating addictive behavior (Koob & Le Moal, 1997).

Because the attentional training inherent in mindfulness meditation had been classically conceptualized as a means of de-automatization (i.e., undoing automaticity; see Deikman, 1966), and mindfulness meditation appeared to be an efficacious means of stress reduction (Kabat-Zinn, 1982), it seemed likely that mindfulness would be effective for treating addictive behavior. But, I suspected that mindfulness alone might be insufficient for producing long-term addiction recovery—a process centered on reclaiming meaning in life (see the "Recovery Enhancement" section below). Similarly, I thought mindfulness alone might not fully remediate the reward system deficit underpinning addiction. Clinical wisdom, cognitive science, and modern neurobiology suggested the need for additional therapeutic techniques, including *reappraisal*, the process of reframing the meaning of adverse life events, and *savoring*, the process of appreciating and amplifying positive life experiences. I began to weave these techniques together in my primary care-based integrative medicine practice working with adults and adolescents suffering from a wide array of mental health problems, substance use disorders, chronic pain conditions, and psychosomatic complaints. As an outgrowth of my training in clinical hypnosis, I knew that indirect suggestion could facilitate access to profound alterations in one's state of consciousness, leading to a significant restructuring of associations and reorganization of the patient's inner life (Erickson, Rossi, & Rossi, 1976). As such, I began to use indirect suggestion to potentiate my delivery and processing of mindfulness, reappraisal, and savoring techniques. Patients who had previously struggled to practice mindfulness through more traditional routes of meditation instruction began to report having great success with the method I was developing. Some of these patients reported becoming better able to see the stressors in their lives as opportunities for psychological growth, and others reported a greater sense of fulfillment and meaning in life. Still others reported experiencing transitory flashes of self-transcendence, where their normal sense of self, typically caught in the trap of pain or addiction, was momentarily eclipsed by a spacious, open, and clear state of awareness, blissful and free from suffering. These early clinical successes let me know I was on the right track in developing this new treatment approach.

Building upon what I was learning from the "living laboratory" of my clinical practice and my study of contemplative wisdom traditions, in 2008 I received a Francisco J. Varela Award from the Mind and Life Institute to develop and test MORE as an intervention for people in inpatient treatment for alcohol use disorder. Results from this pilot trial suggested that MORE might reduce addictive behavior by modifying addiction attentional bias and increasing autonomic recovery from stress and addiction-related cues (Garland, Gaylord, et al., 2010). Given these promising mechanistic findings, in 2009 I began testing MORE in a 5-year Stage 3 randomized controlled trial (RCT) at the same treatment facility: a long-term therapeutic community that served a large number of formerly homeless Black, White, and Latino men with histories of incarceration, addiction, trauma, and psychiatric disorders. In this study, associated with a grant from SAMHSA, MORE was found to outperform both CBT and usual addictions care on multiple mental health and addiction-related outcomes (Garland, Roberts-Lewis, et al., 2016). Before the completion of this trial, I met a physician colleague who encouraged me to combine my clinical experience providing mind–body therapies for chronic pain with my research focus on addiction. I took his advice. Although my colleagues and I have continued to study MORE as a treatment for a wide array of addictive behaviors (e.g., smoking cessation, internet addiction, obesity), the majority of the next 15 years of research on MORE focused on studying the therapy as a treatment for opioid misuse, OUD, and chronic pain.

In 2011, when the opioid crisis was beginning to reach an early peak, I was awarded an R03 grant from the National Institute on Drug Abuse (NIDA) to test a modified version of MORE as a treatment for opioid misuse among people with chronic pain being treated with long-term opioid analgesics. In this Stage 2 RCT, MORE led to clinically significant reductions in chronic pain symptoms, opioid misuse, and craving (Garland et al., 2014). In fact, MORE was twice as powerful as standard supportive group psychotherapy in reducing the occurrence of opioid misuse symptoms consistent with having an OUD diagnosis. My colleagues and I also made a number of mechanistic discoveries with data from this trial. We found that MORE reduced automatic attentional bias and improved cognitive control under conditions of stress (Garland, Baker, et al., 2017; Garland, Bryan, et al., 2019; Garland & Howard, 2013). We also found that MORE increased positive emotion regulation; patients in MORE had 2.75 times the odds of those in supportive psychotherapy to be able to increase or maintain positive moods from moment to moment in everyday life (Garland, Bryan, Finan, et al., 2017). Most notably, we found that the effects of MORE on reducing opioid craving and opioid misuse were associated with a restructuring of reward processing from valuing drug-related rewards back to valuing natural rewards, as indicated by electroencephalography (EEG; Garland, Froeliger, et al., 2015b) and autonomic measures (Garland et al., 2014; Garland, Howard, et al., 2017). In 2015, a pilot study of MORE as a treatment for smoking cessation found similar evidence of restructuring reward processing via functional magnetic resonance imaging measures of brain reward system function (Froeliger et al., 2017). Taken together, these data suggested the allostatic process of addiction might be reversed by teaching people how to savor natural healthy rewards—a signal discovery in the history of MORE (and the treatment of addiction, for that matter) that led me to catalyze my *restructuring reward hypothesis*: Shifting valuation from drug-related rewards back to valuing natural rewards will reduce craving and addictive behavior (Garland, 2016, 2021).

As a result of these discoveries, I realized savoring was an exceptionally important component of MORE. So I began to strengthen this aspect of the program by embedding an implicit emphasis on savoring throughout, in addition to the explicit savoring training session. I also began to perfect the MORE approach to teaching mindfulness and other mind–body skills. After listening to hundreds of hours of tapes of therapists delivering MORE, I began to distill the basic processes integral to helping patients successfully consolidate what they had learned from their practice of mind–body skills during the MORE sessions and to generalize that learning to coping with symptoms of pain, distress, and opioid misuse in everyday life. These insights ultimately blossomed into the PURER (phenomenology, utilization, reframing, education/expectancy, and reinforcement) processing approach described in Chapter 5.

As a result of the clinical and mechanistic research findings from our preliminary studies, in 2016 my colleagues and I were awarded two major, multiyear, federal research grants: an R01 grant from NIDA to conduct a definitive efficacy test of MORE as a treatment for chronic pain and opioid misuse in civilians, as well as a clinical trial award from the U.S. Department of Defense's Congressionally Directed Medical Research Program to test MORE for the same indication in U.S. veterans and military personnel. These studies became the central focus of my clinical research program for the latter half of the decade and were instrumental in the continued development of the MORE program.

While these studies were in progress, I continued to investigate the therapeutic mechanisms of MORE. In 2019, I conducted a second Stage 2 RCT of MORE for people with chronic pain who were prescribed opioids but who had not yet progressed to opioid misuse (Garland, Hanley, Riquino, et al., 2019), and found that MORE reduced opioid misuse risk by decreasing pain and enhancing a range of positive psychological functions, including positive emotions, savoring, meaning in life, and self-transcendence—the sense of being connected to something greater than the self. This was the first evidence in the scientific literature that a relatively brief mindfulness therapy could elicit self-transcendent experiences, and that increasing self-transcendence had important clinical consequences. This discovery led us to optimize MORE by including a greater focus on self-transcendence during PURER and developing additional session material aimed at stimulating self-transcendent experiences (see Chapter 7). Also in this study we found that MORE decreased opioid dosing by 32%, and the effects of MORE on reducing opioid dose were explained in part by increased autonomic self-regulation during mindfulness meditation (Garland et al., 2020). This was the first time we directly tied a key clinical outcome to the state of mindfulness as cultivated during the foundational MORE meditation practice.

At the same time, we embarked upon a major series of mechanistic experiments and found additional evidence for the restructuring reward hypothesis across four studies of MORE. Specifically, we found MORE decreased EEG responses to drug cues while enhancing EEG responses to natural reward cues during savoring. In addition, we found that the effects of MORE on reducing opioid misuse were mediated by increases in positive emotional responses to natural healthy rewards (Garland, Atchley, et al., 2019). These data represented the first finding in the scientific literature from an RCT that an MBI could reduce drug cue–reactivity in the brain—a completely novel finding with major significance to the science of addiction. At the same time, my colleague Adam Hanley and I found that MORE led to a sevenfold increase in the ratio of pleasant to unpleasant sensations in the body (Hanley & Garland, 2019a). Then, a little over a year later, we found MORE increased frontal midline theta EEG oscillations during meditation that were associated with increased reports of self-transcendence and decreased opioid use over time (Hudak et al., 2021). Most recently, in another mechanistic trial, we replicated earlier findings showing that MORE increases EEG responses to natural rewards, brain changes that were linked with an improved ability to experience healthy pleasure in everyday life (Garland, Fix, et al., 2023).

As we awaited completion of the full-scale clinical trial of MORE, my colleagues and I launched a pilot study funded by the National Center for Complementary and Integrative Health to test

> MORE aims to restructure reward processing in the brain.

MORE as an adjunct to methadone treatment for people with OUD and chronic pain. In a highly racially diverse, urban sample, we found that MORE led to significantly greater decreases in days of opioid use, other drug use, craving, pain, and depression than methadone treatment as usual (Cooperman et al., 2021). Furthermore, we found that MORE decreased the intensity of opioid craving in everyday life by about 50%, and the effects of MORE on decreasing craving were linked with increases in momentary positive emotions (Garland, Hanley, Kline, et al., 2019), again providing support for the restructuring reward hypothesis.

In 2021, we completed the NIDA R01-funded clinical trial of MORE, and obtained conclusive evidence of MORE's efficacy as a treatment for chronic pain and opioid misuse (Garland, Hanley, Nakamura, et al., 2022). In this trial, we enrolled 250 patients with chronic pain, all of whom were showing signs of opioid misuse at the beginning of the study. Before the trial began, patients reported a mean pain level of 5.5 out of 10, and were taking on average about 100 morphine milligram equivalents a day. At baseline, nearly 70% of patients met criteria for major depressive disorder, and 62% met criteria for full-blown OUD. Nine months after completion of the study treatments, MORE had reduced opioid misuse by 45%, nearly tripling the effect of standard supportive therapy. MORE also significantly reduced opioid use through the 9-month follow-up, and 36% of patients were able to cut their opioid dose in half or greater. In addition, MORE significantly reduced chronic pain symptoms, with 58% of patients reporting clinically meaningful decreases in pain-related functional impairment. MORE also had robust antidepressant effects and led to clinically significant decreases in posttraumatic stress symptoms. At the same time, MORE significantly increased positive emotions, a sense of meaning in life, and self-transcendence, with these effects maintained 9 months later. In addition to treating their symptoms of pain and opioid misuse, MORE had helped the patients become happier people in general—attesting to the life-altering impacts of this therapeutic approach.

Then, in 2022, we completed the U.S. Department of Defense-funded clinical trial (Garland, Nakamura, et al., 2024). In a sample of 230 veterans and active duty military personnel who had been in pain an average of 20 years, we again found that MORE led to statistically significant reductions in chronic pain and opioid dosing through an 8-month follow-up. Patients in MORE were able to reduce their opioid use by 21%, on average. MORE also significantly decreased opioid craving and opioid attentional bias, while reducing anhedonia and increasing positive emotions. These findings replicated our NIH R01-funded study of MORE, providing additional strong support for MORE's efficacy in a second, independent, full-scale RCT.

That same year, we completed the largest neuroscientific study of mindfulness as a treatment for addiction ever conducted (Garland, Hanley, Hudak, et al., 2022). We replicated our earlier results (Hudak et al., 2021) by showing that the effects of MORE on reducing opioid misuse through a 9-month follow-up were mediated by increases in frontal midline theta EEG activity during mindfulness meditation. Frontal midline theta is a well-known biomarker of cognitive control, but it increases during states of flow, when the sense of self is suspended and transcended during deep cognitive absorption with ongoing activity. Thus, mindfulness-induced self-transcendence was associated with a brain signature of self-control with clear anti-addictive properties. Replicating these results across two RCTs with two independent samples indicates that we may have indeed found a key mechanism by which mindfulness reduces addictive behavior.

Most recently, in 2023, we completed a full-scale clinical trial of MORE for people with OUD and chronic pain (Cooperman et al., 2023). In this study, we examined the efficacy of MORE as delivered online by telehealth in a highly racially diverse, low-income sample of 154 patients receiving methadone treatment at addiction clinics in an urban area of New Jersey. Patients treated with the telehealth MORE intervention showed a significantly lower rate of relapse back to drug use, significantly fewer days of drug use, lower chronic pain symptoms, and less depression relative to patients who received a standard addictions treatment approach. These data suggest that MORE is accessible to a wide range of people from varying socioeconomic and education levels, and that this novel therapeutic approach can substantially improve addiction treatment outcomes.

To date, MORE's efficacy across a wide range of patients has been supported by 12 RCTs and two meta-analyses (Li et al., 2021; Parisi et al., 2022). Of these trials, six RCTs involving more than 800 patients clearly demonstrate that MORE is an efficacious treatment for treating chronic pain, opioid misuse, and OUD. In light of this body of evidence, I felt it was now time to disseminate MORE to clinicians and patients in the real world.

Mindfulness

Though the concept of mindfulness will be expanded upon throughout this book, this term deserves a brief introduction here. *Mindfulness* is an English word for a range of concepts and techniques that emerged in Asia millennia ago in multiple Buddhist, Hindu, Yogic, and Taoist traditions, but also has parallels in the mystical branches of Judaism, Christianity, and Islam, as well as in the shamanic practices of multiple indigenous cultures around the world. Acknowledging and drawing upon these ancient contemplative roots, the entire MORE approach is oriented toward and grounded in a secular form of mindfulness practice that began to be integrated into health care 4 decades ago (Kabat-Zinn, 1982).

In the modern parlance of psychology and neuroscience, the term *mindfulness* has applied to both a set of mental training practices (i.e., meditation techniques), as well as to the mental states and traits cultivated by these practices. Simply put, mindfulness is the process of observing and accepting present-moment thoughts, emotions, sensations, and perceptions from the perspective of a witness, while reflecting back upon of the field of awareness in which those mental contents arise. This meta-awareness, or "awareness of awareness," is a critical aspect of mindfulness. On the one hand, the capacity to be mindful is a basic property of the human mind resting in its natural state. On the other hand, with disciplined practice, mindfulness may deepen over time such that for brief moments the normal sense of one's self as separate from the world begins to fade, leaving a profound sense of expansive wholeness or pure consciousness in its wake (Metzinger, 2024). In those self-transcendent moments, "Mind is like space; it has the nature of space; equal to space, it encompasses everything" (Namgyal, 2006, p. 192).

> Mindfulness is the practice of observing and accepting present-moment thoughts, emotions, sensations, and perceptions, and witnessing them unfold in the field of awareness.

How then is the concept of mindfulness, whether as the mind's basic nature or a rarified state of consciousness, related to the treatment of people suffering from chronic pain and problematic opioid use? Chapter 3 provides a detailed theoretical response to this question. To summarize here, chronic pain, opioid misuse, and OUD are all conditions that are often preserved and exacerbated by maladaptive mental habits—for instance, feeling helpless to cope with pain, or fixating on thoughts about the next dose of opioids. These unhelpful patterns of attending, thinking, and reacting often occur in spite of the patient's well-intentioned effort to control them due to the process of automaticity—that is, they sometimes occur autonomously and unconsciously, against the patient's will. In this sense, these automatic, maladaptive mental habits operate in a context of *mindlessness*. Given the role that mindlessness plays in perpetuating pain and addictive behavior, a treatment oriented around mindfulness is a logical solution to these prevalent and pernicious problems. Through mindfulness, automatic habits can be deautomatized—that is, they can be surfaced in awareness, brought under conscious control, and thereby transformed.

Recovery Enhancement

At the outset, it is important to emphasize MORE's focus on *recovery enhancement* as distinguished from *relapse prevention*. The goal of relapse prevention is to help patients maintain abstinence from substance use by teaching them skills to cope with high-risk situations where relapse is likely (Marlatt & Donovan, 2005). In contrast, *recovery* may be defined as "a process of change through which individuals improve their health and wellness, live a self-directed life, and strive to reach their full potential" (SAMHSA, 2011). In this sense, recovery is a holistic process that attends to the multiple dimensions of hedonic and eudaimonic well-being, extending far beyond abstinence from drug use. Furthermore, the recovery perspective regards lapses back to drug use as part of the normative developmental pathway in which a person using substances eventually reaches a state of optimal functioning. This consideration is particularly appropriate for individuals with chronic pain who have been prescribed long-term opioid therapy, who, due to their medical condition, may remain taking opioids for the rest of their lives. Here, the goal is harm reduction (i.e., reduced opioid overuse or misuse, as well as prevention of the negative sequelae of that use), not abstinence. At the same time, the recovery perspective involves an ethos of optimism: the belief that given enough time and coping resources, people can heal from physical and emotional pain, and ultimately, liberate themselves from destructive habits. MORE was designed to enhance the recovery process for people striving to overcome addiction. MORE is philosophically grounded in this recovery-enhancement perspective, and built upon the belief in the inherent capacity of individuals to transcend and transform their limitations into opportunities for growth and meaning making. This philosophical perspective permeates MORE and serves as the living core of the intervention from which its many concepts and techniques radiate.

   Thus, from the perspective underlying MORE, a person suffering from chronic pain, emotional distress, and problematic opioid use has, like all human beings, the innate resilience and "basic goodness" (Trungpa, 1985) needed to access an inner wellspring of well-being that transcends the travails and tragedies of life. However, this radical transformation from viewing oneself as deficient and broken to experiencing oneself as full of basic goodness does not occur through magic—it develops from the repeated and incremental practice of adopting salutogenic ways of thinking and behaving in the world, day after day, moment by moment. Each time a person intentionally challenges negative mental states and cultivates positive ones, the process of recovery advances toward its ultimate end goal of inner awakening and self-liberation (Teasdale, 2022). MORE is founded on this foundational recovery perspective pointing to the possibility of transformation through training. MORE is, at its core, a system of mental training aimed at enhancing flourishing and meaning in life amid the endless cycles of suffering and joy that characterize human existence.

Because mindfulness is, at heart, an experiential rather than conceptual process, it is necessary for you, as a MORE therapist, to develop your own disciplined mindfulness practice. There is no better way to come to understand mindfulness than through the practice of mindfulness itself. Chapter 3 provides some recommendations in that regard. In addition to having their own personal practice of mindfulness, MORE therapists should aim to cultivate attitudes of compassion and empowerment toward their patients, as described in the next section.

Ethical Values Underlying MORE: Compassion and Empowerment as the Foundations of Healing

Before embarking upon a description of the scientific and theoretical synthesis underlying the MORE program, I would like to speak to the ethical values foundational to its authentic and successful implementation. First and foremost, the MORE therapist should have compassion for their patient. It is easy to become judgmental, to blame the patient for having a "victim stance" or a "personality disorder," or suggest the client is exaggerating their painful symptoms by "somaticizing" or "catastrophizing." So too, the labels of "drug seeker" and "addict" are unfortunately a part of the common lexicon in health care. These clinical labels stigmatize the patient (Slade et al., 2009), drive a wedge between clinician and client, undermine the development of an authentic therapeutic relationship (itself a precondition to effective MORE therapy), and belie the true anguish of chronic pain. Though the experience of pain may or may not be directly proportional to tissue damage, the potential lack of a nociceptive basis for a given patient's pain does not in any way diminish the suffering that person is experiencing. Someone who has not experienced pain for months, years, or decades on end has difficulty appreciating the terrible impact of such an experience. Chronic pain is demoralizing, dis-spiriting, fatiguing, and can rob a person of their sense of self, their very identity (Armentrout, 1979). Indeed, when someone who has lived a life full of vigorous, athletic activity experiences an accident resulting in severe and debilitating back pain, and then has trouble walking up the street, picking up their young children, or carrying groceries from the car, this can erode the sense of being a man, a woman, a husband or wife, a parent, or a capable person. Imagine what it is like to experience such a loss of self. Imagine what it is like to have your every waking thought and concern bent toward the sense that your own body was betraying you. Imagine what it is like to have your attention inexorably drawn toward sensations of stabbing, searing, cutting, gripping, aching, and burning for what seems like every minute of every day.

This kind of suffering goes far beyond physical pain—it can be heartbreaking. To help someone suffering from pain, one must adopt a stance of compassion toward that person, accepting the reality of their suffering and letting go of judgment and blame. A human being is a biopsychosocial system, embedded in and constituted by larger biopsychosocial systems, and thus an innumerable number of forces impinge upon that being in any given moment to shape one's behavior and internal state (Bateson, 1972; Engel, 1977). So any reductive causal account of that state is bound to be biased and at best only a partial view. We cannot know why the person behaves and feels as they do. Therefore, if we aim to help our client to shift their behavior and internal state, we must accept the reality of their suffering, regardless of its source, and respond to it with empathy (Feldman & Kuyken, 2011). This root of compassionate action is the ethical precondition for effective MORE practice.

Second, the MORE therapist should adopt an empowerment mindset. As just discussed, some people with chronic pain on LTOT come to feel powerless over their conditions. Indeed, the depression that often co-occurs with chronic pain, opioid misuse, and OUD is marked by a sense of learned helplessness and hopelessness—the sense that nothing can be done to make things better. This depressed attitude is understandable, given that many people in this situation have come to believe their bodies have been permanently damaged. They may have been told they suffer from incurable conditions, or that they have mental health disorders caused by faulty brain circuitry or defective genes. Furthermore, many such individuals have had multiple medical procedures, have seen a seemingly endless succession of health care providers, and have tried a veritable pharmacy worth of prescription medications and supplements, with little relief in return. Finally, opioid use (prescribed or illicit) is marked by stigma and shame. Our society labels those who take opioids as prescribed by their physicians as "addicts" and assumes that opioid use implies criminality. No wonder why such individuals feel so disempowered, and judge themselves so harshly.

The empowerment mindset works against that hopelessness and helplessness (Deegan, 1997). It is the idea that one can help oneself, the conditions of a person's life can be improved, and progress can be made, no matter where the starting place. Empowerment begins with the unwavering belief in the individual's capacity to act to transform and heal themselves. Empowerment must be balanced with compassion, for without compassion, this attitude could devolve into victim blaming or the notion that one can pull themselves up by their own bootstraps. In MORE, we first acknowledge that the client has become trapped in a web of forces from which it is difficult to escape, and then we recognize that the client also possesses an untapped wellspring of healing power from which the energy for change, however distant and latent, can be summoned. Thus, in MORE we adopt a nonpathologizing view of the patient. We regard people as resilient survivors, not diagnoses or victims. We believe that no matter the starting place, a person is capable of significant growth and healing, because their true nature is rooted in basic goodness. And we know such growth can emerge only from hard work and from persistent and determined application of mental force, just as the waters of a mountain stream can polish a rough piece of granite into smooth pebbles given enough time, or even carve solid earth into a grand and majestic canyon.

> No matter the starting place, a person is capable of significant growth and healing.

With these dual attitudes of compassion (Lama & Vreeland, 2001) and empowerment (Deegan, 1997), you are ready to embark upon learning how to use MORE to help your patients free themselves from the clutches of chronic pain and addictive behavior. In the next chapter I discuss the complexities of how chronic pain can lead to opioid misuse and OUD.

Chapter 2

The Downward Spiral
from Chronic Pain to Addiction

To appreciate how to use MORE to help patients struggling with chronic pain and opioid-related issues, and for whom MORE is an appropriate treatment, a nuanced understanding of the mechanisms linking chronic pain to opioid misuse and OUD is required. As an anonymous sage once said, "If you want to know how to fix a problem, you've got to know what makes the problem tick." To that end, my colleagues and I developed the downward spiral model (Garland, Froeliger, Zeidan, et al., 2013). This model depicts the destructive processes and maladaptive feedback loops that unwittingly propel a person suffering from prolonged pain down the path toward an eventual loss of control over opioid use. I have been studying these risk mechanisms undergirding opioid misuse and OUD in people with chronic pain for more than a decade, and the discoveries my colleagues and I have made, along with many other great scientific insights from the field, informed the development of MORE. This chapter first discusses the types of patients who are appropriate for treatment with MORE, and then details the downward spiral model linking chronic pain to opioid misuse and OUD (see Figure 2.1) to provide a comprehensive understanding of why such patients are struggling.

Identification of Problematic Opioid Use

Before discussing the indications and contraindications for MORE and detailing the downward spiral model, we need to define diagnostic categories to classify opioid use patterns and their bio-psychosocial consequences. *Long-term opioid therapy* is defined as the use of prescription opioids to alleviate physical pain for a period of 90 consecutive days or longer (Chou et al., 2009). While LTOT in and of itself does not indicate addiction, it confers multiple health risks associated with addiction, including the development of opioid misuse, OUD, and overdose (Chou et al., 2015). (For the American Psychiatric Association's [2013] current description and criteria for OUD, see page 541 of the *Diagnostic and Statistical Manual of Mental Disorders, Fifth Edition*.) It should be noted that for people who are prescribed opioids for chronic pain, tolerance and withdrawal do

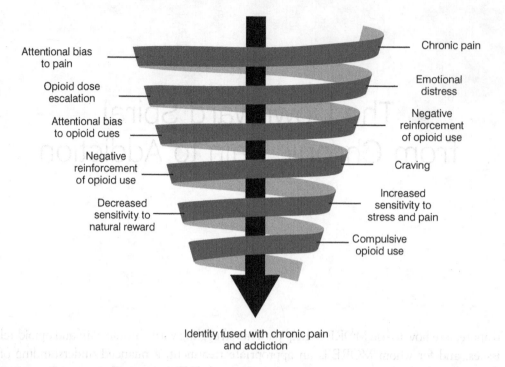

FIGURE 2.1. Downward spiral of chronic pain, opioid misuse, and addiction. From "The Downward Spiral of Chronic Pain, Prescription Opioid Misuse, and Addiction" by E. L. Garland, B. Froeliger, F. Zeidan, K. Partin, and M. O. Howard. Copyright © 2013 Elsevier. Adapted by permission.

not constitute criteria for OUD, given that the majority of people on LTOT show opioid tolerance and would experience withdrawal upon running out of medication; yet neither of these symptoms necessarily indicates the loss of control over opioid use or compulsive opioid use that is characteristic of OUD. However, OUD may be presaged by the presence of *opioid misuse* behaviors, such as taking higher doses of opioids than prescribed, using opioids for reasons other than pain (e.g., to get high or to alleviate negative emotions like sadness, fear, or anger), obtaining opioid prescriptions from multiple providers (i.e., "doctor shopping"), or obtaining opioids from the street (Butler et al., 2006, 2007; Ives et al., 2006). The presence of more serious misuse behaviors may mark the transition from sanctioned use of opioids to development of full-blown OUD. Opioid misuse is more prevalent than OUD. In 2022, 8.5 million Americans misused prescription opioids, and 6.5 million had an OUD (SAMHSA, 2023). Although rates of misuse decreased modestly when the Centers for Disease Control opioid prescription guidelines were released in 2016 (Dowell et al., 2016), they increased again under COVID-19, and opioid misuse and addiction remain a significant problem in society.

Assessing Patients for Their Appropriateness for MORE

Before embarking upon delivering the MORE intervention, we need to understand whether MORE is the right fit for a given patient. When assessing patients for MORE, consideration should be given to where along the progression from LTOT to opioid misuse and OUD the patient may fall, as well as to the patient's readiness to change and the presence of safety issues that may be a contraindication for treatment.

The first category of patient who may be appropriate for MORE is the patient who has been prescribed opioids for a chronic pain condition, and who takes their opioid medication as prescribed, but is unsatisfied by the degree of pain relief they have achieved. This type of patient might also be seeking assistance in coping with the emotional distress associated with chronic pain and its impact on functioning. Alternatively, the patient might be seeking help to reduce their opioid dose or to taper off opioids completely. Tapering is often initiated by the prescribing physician, but sometimes patients themselves wish to reduce their opioid use. In either case, tapering should be monitored by a physician and done slowly to minimize withdrawal symptoms (~10% reduction in dose per month) according to best-practice guidelines (Rubin, 2019) in a patient-centered manner that preserves patient agency and positive expectancy (Darnall & Fields, 2022).

The second category of patient who may especially benefit from MORE is the patient who may be misusing opioids that were originally prescribed to alleviate chronic pain. This type of patient might present similarly to someone adhering to their prescribed LTOT regimen in the sense that they may be seeking help to alleviate unsuccessfully treated pain or emotional distress. Often, such patients are reluctant to disclose opioid misuse behaviors. Opioid misuse may be inferred by signs of emotional volatility, allegedly poor response to opioid medication, expressing a preference for certain types of opioid medication, running out of opioid medication early, seeking opioid prescriptions from multiple health care providers, multiple emergency room visits, and signs and symptoms of intoxication during a clinical interview. It should be noted that there are few direct measures of opioid misuse. Drug urine screens cannot be used to detect misuse of prescription opioids because they provide only qualitative (e.g., "Did the patient use opioids?") and not quantitative readouts of opioid use (e.g., "What dose did the patient take?"). However, urine screens can detect the presence of nonprescribed opioids and illicit substances that, when taken in combination with the prescribed opioid, constitute opioid misuse.

Statewide prescription drug monitoring programs can verify whether patients have been receiving opioid prescriptions from multiple providers, but these data are often inaccessible to behavioral health providers. In the absence of objective measures of misuse, various assessment tools for opioid misuse have been published, including the Current Opioid Misuse Measure (Butler et al., 2007), the Addiction Behaviors Checklist (Wu et al., 2006), and the Opioid Compliance Checklist (Jamison et al., 2016). All have their strengths and limitations. Self-reporting of opioid misuse can be encouraged through careful and compassionate interviewing skills. Normalizing behaviors like opioid dose escalation (e.g., "Many patients feel that their doctor hasn't prescribed a high enough opioid dose, so they sometimes decide to take a little extra to take the edge off their pain") or self-medication of negative emotions with opioids (e.g., "Often, people find that opioids not only relieve pain but also reduce stress or bad feelings. I wonder if you can relate to that") can help patients to open up about their misuse of opioids. Assurances of confidentiality and expressions of nonjudgment can be extremely helpful (e.g., "I'm not here to judge you, I'm here to help. I understand that not everyone takes opioids exactly as they were prescribed by their doctor").

Like patients who take opioids as prescribed, those who misuse opioids may be seeking your help to reduce their opioid dose, or to stop using opioids entirely. Or they may be undergoing opioid tapering and need help coping with the consequent withdrawal and distress. In either case, a subtle motivational enhancement approach may be needed to work successfully with these patients, many of whom do not recognize they are misusing opioids and do not identify with engaging in addictive behavior. This motivational approach is embedded in the MORE treatment sequence. In brief, MORE attempts to "meet the patient where they are" by first providing techniques to alleviate chronic pain and emotional distress. Rather than directly confronting patients about their opioid use or exhorting them to change, patients are asked to bring mindful awareness to their opioid use patterns. With each successive session, more detailed attention is given to patient reports of opioid use patterns that may be reflective of misuse. After patients begin to experience relief and motivation for engaging in the MORE practices increases, the concept of craving is introduced in the fifth session, after which patients are encouraged to look at their opioid use from this lens, and to consider changing their opioid use patterns.

But there is a third category of patient who may seek your help: the patient with chronic pain *and* OUD. This patient may already be receiving OUD treatment in the form of an MOUD, like buprenorphine or methadone, or the patient may have an untreated OUD but be experiencing severe social, occupational, or legal consequences for their opioid use. We

> Understand the patient's history with opioid use, and their reasons for seeking help.

have found that patients with OUD are in some ways more open to treatment than those who misuse opioids but have not yet progressed to OUD, in the sense that they often recognize that they have a problematic pattern of opioid use that requires active change efforts on their part. On the other hand, these patients may have lost control over their opioid use and be engaging in compulsive opioid use against their best intentions. Furthermore, their lives may be highly unstable, insofar as such patients are often facing severe social and economic issues, including job loss, homelessness, institutionalization, and incarceration. These challenges may present barriers to treatment with MORE. Nonetheless, such patients are often seeking help to adhere to their MOUD and to keep from relapsing back to opioid use. Or, they may be stable on MOUD but still experiencing untreated chronic pain and emotional distress. Finally, their opioid use may be out of control, and they may be unwilling to use MOUD to treat their addiction, but open to receiving a behavioral therapy like MORE. MORE can be useful for any of these patients.

Given the wide range of patient presentations appropriate for MORE, the MORE treatment manual portion of this book (Sessions 1–8) includes language addressing prescribed opioid use, opioid misuse, and opioid addiction. However, keep in mind that such language may be inappropriate, stigmatizing, or off-putting to patients who are at different stages of opioid use. For instance, talking about addiction, craving, and recovery may be offensive to patients who take opioids as prescribed by their physicians. In that case, you as the therapist should tailor the language in the treatment manual to omit or reframe concepts that might clinically be irrelevant or offend the patient. Yet, discussion of addiction, craving, and recovery might be informative or serve a prevention function for a patient who has not yet progressed to opioid misuse or OUD. On the other hand, talking about issues with prescription opioid analgesics like oxycodone might not be the best fit for a patient with OUD who is now being treated with methadone. When in doubt, and if you have a mixed group of patients, you can always offer a disclaimer like

"What I'm about to say might not fit your situation perfectly. I'm not trying to offend you. If what I am talking about doesn't seem to match your situation well, feel free to let me know, and we can shift gears a bit. That said, you might find you can learn something from this content even if you aren't struggling with this exact issue."

As a MORE therapist, you will have to use your clinical judgment and knowledge of the patient's stage of opioid use and readiness to change in order to decide which language is appropriate to share in which context.

Safety Issues That May Be Contraindications for MORE

In the many research studies that have been done on MORE, my colleagues and I have included patients struggling with a wide array of chronic medical conditions and serious psychiatric disorders, including major depressive disorder, generalized anxiety disorder, posttraumatic stress disorder (PTSD), somatization disorder, and substance use disorders. We have also included patients with bipolar disorder who are stabilized on medication and have not exhibited recent manic episodes. However, due to research ethics considerations we have excluded patients with active suicidal intent and psychosis from our trials. Whether MORE is safe and beneficial for such patients remains to be seen. That said, we have included many patients with a moderate degree of suicidal ideation in our studies, and given the strong antidepressant effects of MORE (Garland, Hanley, Nakamura, et al., 2022), MORE is likely to ease suicidal thoughts and feelings. If the patient is willing to contract for safety and has no suicidal intent or recent attempts, they are probably appropriate for MORE. Given meta-analyses demonstrating the safety and positive effects of MBIs for psychosis and schizophrenia (Jansen et al., 2020; Louise et al., 2018), it is also possible that MORE could benefit such patients, but until rigorous clinical trial data are collected, caution is warranted.

MORE may be useful for patients experiencing acute opioid withdrawal, though empirical data on this topic are lacking. When, on occasion, patients have reported withdrawal symptoms coincident with their participation in the 8-week MORE program, the mindfulness of pain practice in MORE (detailed in Session 2) has been useful in easing withdrawal symptoms in much the same way that it eases physical pain. Be aware that if your patient is experiencing withdrawal, their cognitive faculties may be compromised as they suffer with physical discomfort, and so due to reduced concentration they may need shorter meditation sessions and more support and positive reinforcement through the treatment process.

Finally, it should be noted that patients do not need to abstain from opioid or other substance use during treatment with MORE. MORE is undergirded by a harm reduction perspective—we are ready to meet the patient "where they are" in terms of their readiness to change and assume that some benefit can be derived, even for patients who are mildly intoxicated during sessions. Given that most patients will be taking a prescription opioid on a near daily basis when they participate in MORE sessions, they may on occasion appear sedated or groggy during the session, depending on the proximity of the last opioid dose to the session time. In our experience, patients in this state may still receive some benefit from participating in the session. Because severe, acute substance

> MORE does not require abstinence from opioids or other drugs.

intoxication may lead to disruptive behavior, patients who show signs of being very high may need to be asked to leave MORE group sessions and return the following week when they are in better shape to participate.

Pain as a Biopsychosocial Phenomenon

The downward spiral of behavioral escalation from a patient's first opioid prescription to LTOT, opioid misuse, and OUD begins with chronic pain (see Figure 2.1). Therefore, a detailed account of pain is needed.

Pain is a complex, biopsychosocial phenomenon that arises from the interaction of multiple brain and body systems with cognitive, affective, and interpersonal processes. The International Association for the Study of Pain has offered the following definition of pain: "An unpleasant sensory and emotional experience associated with, or resembling that associated with, actual or potential tissue damage" (Raja et al., 2020). A quick read of this authoritative definition clearly reveals that pain is not merely physical but also involves mental components, including emotions, thoughts, and expectations—for example, the anticipation of future harm. Also, pain does not require "actual tissue damage," since it can also occur with the sensory and emotional experience resembling potential tissue damage. In other words, believing that one's body has been damaged can cause pain, even if no such damage has occurred.

> Pain is not merely physical, but also involves emotions, thoughts, and expectations.

Take, for example, the case of a 29-year-old construction worker (Dimsdale & Dantzer, 2007). He was admitted to the emergency room howling in pain from a 7-inch nail that had pierced all the way through his steel-toed boot and was protruding from the other side. He required high doses of intravenous morphine in order to calm him down enough so that his boot could be removed. And when the boot had been removed, the patient and medical personnel were shocked to see the nail had passed through the space between two of his toes without puncturing his skin! No damage had actually occurred, but rather the expectation of tissue damage caused serious pain. On the other hand, take the case of the gentleman who came to the dentist complaining of a mild toothache (Dimsdale & Dantzer, 2007). Upon receiving an X-ray, both he and his dentist were appalled to discover that a large nail from his nail gun had shot through his nostril and had pierced his skull—an event that had occurred completely outside his awareness. In this case there was massive tissue damage, but almost no pain!

How are we to understand such bizarre phenomena? To begin to grasp how events like this are even possible, we need to understand the role that the brain plays in constructing the experience of pain.

The Biology of Pain

Pain Processing in the Nervous System

When noxious stimuli (i.e., mechanical [being pierced by a nail], thermal [touching a hot stove], or chemical [a snake's venom] stimuli that can damage tissue) impinge upon the body, information about the damaging impact of these stimuli on bodily tissues is transmitted through the peripheral nervous system to the central and autonomic nervous systems. This transmission of information about actual tissue damage (or the potential for such damage, should the noxious stimulus continue to be applied) to the brain is known as *nociception* (Julius & Basbaum, 2001). Specialized nerve receptors known as nociceptors attached to thin myelinated Aδ and unmyelinated C fibers carry this information to the dorsal horn of the spine from the damaged body part (Brodal, 2004). Although usually transmission of nociceptive information results in pain perception, nociception can occur in the absence of awareness of pain (the nail-in-nose story above), and pain can occur in the absence of measurably noxious stimuli (the nail-in-boot story above). This dissociation between nociception and pain is observable in instances of massive trauma (such as in battlefield injuries) when victims exhibit a stoic painless state in order to focus on survival despite severe injury, and conversely, when people with functional pain syndromes (e.g., fibromyalgia, irritable bowel syndrome) report considerable anguish in spite of having no observable tissue damage.

Pain perception (Dubin & Patapoutian, 2010; Loeser & Melzack, 1999) is a subjective experience that occurs with actual or potential damage to the body. The experience of pain is often undergirded by nociception. Nociception is processed by two neural processing receptors: fast-acting Aδ fibers that produce the experience of a sharp, prickling pain, and slower C fibers that produce a dull, throbbing, aching, burning pain. These pain experiences occur in two phases during and after an acute injury, although these phases may be difficult to differentiate subjectively (Bishop & Landau, 1958). The first phase, which is not extremely unpleasant, occurs within several hundred milliseconds of exposure to the painful stimulus and is known as fast pain. The second phase, known as slow pain, is more unpleasant, less localized, and occurs after a delay of 1–2 seconds after injury.

Nociceptive information is carried along the axons of peripheral nerves that terminate in the dorsal horn of the spine. From the dorsal horn, messages are relayed up the spinal cord and through the spinothalamic tract to the thalamus. The thalamus serves as the "gate" or the "relay station" for sensory information to the cerebral cortex (Sherman & Guillery, 1996). From the thalamus, nociception is relayed, in feedback loops, to various cortical and subcortical brain regions, including the amygdala, hypothalamus, periaqueductal grey, basal ganglia, and regions of cerebral cortex (Willis & Westlund, 1997). It is here in the cortex and the limbic system where nociception is translated into the conscious experience of pain. For instance, when nociceptors are stimulated by noxious stimuli, the somatosensory cortex, the insula, and the anterior cingulate cortex become activated, and activation in these brain regions is correlated with the subjective experience of pain (Tracey & Mantyh, 2007).

Molecular Mediators of Pain

Nociception involves a flow of molecular messengers in the peripheral and central nervous systems. When activated by a noxious stimulus, nociceptors transmit the "damage signal" via the excitatory neurotransmitter glutamate (Petrenko et al., 2003). At the same time, an "inflammatory soup" comprising chemicals such as proinflammatory cytokines (e.g., IL-1β), peptides (e.g., bradykinin, substance P), neurotransmitters (e.g., serotonin), lipids (e.g., prostaglandins), and neurotrophins (e.g., nerve growth factor) is released at the site of the injury (Loeser & Melzack, 1999).

As a result of these neurochemical changes in the local environment of nociceptors, the activation of Aδ and C fibers increases, and pain is amplified (Besson, 1999).

As nociceptive information is transmitted up the spinothalamic tract, norepinephrine (i.e., adrenaline) is released from locus coeruleus projections to the thalamus, which relays nociceptive information to the somatosensory cortex, hypothalamus, and hippocampus (Voisin et al., 2005; Yaksh, 1985). To regulate this influx of nociceptive input, the brain secretes endogenous opioids like beta-endorphin and enkephalin, which inhibit pain processing in the nervous system (Basbaum & Fields, 1984; Yaksh, 1987). Opioid drugs (e.g., morphine, oxycodone, heroin) also stimulate these same opioid receptors to produce analgesia, but chronic exposure to opioids can down-regulate the opioid receptors, making them less sensitive to opioids (i.e., tolerance), and affecting the release of endogenous opioids in the brain (Christie, 2008). A number of other neurochemicals are also involved in pain perception, but there is no need to further elaborate on the complex neuropharmacology of nociception and central-peripheral pain modulation here.

Central Modulation of Pain

At the same time, the brain does not passively receive nociceptive information from the body. Instead, the brain actively regulates nociception by modulating activity at the dorsal horn of the spine via descending projections from the cortex and the limbic system through the medulla (Melzack & Wall, 1965). The descending pain modulatory system provides a physiological means for the central nervous system to select which nociceptive signals from the spinal cord enter into awareness.

The descending pain modulatory system consists of cortical, subcortical, and brain stem structures, including the prefrontal cortex, anterior cingulate cortex, insula, amygdala, hypothalamus, periaqueductal grey, rostral ventromedial medulla, and dorsolateral pons/tegmentum. Reynolds (1969) first observed that directly stimulating the periaqueductal grey with electricity could produce potent analgesic effects as shown by the ability to endure major surgery without pain. But mental experiences can also modulate pain through this system. For instance, exerting cognitive control to cope by distracting attention away from pain activates the prefrontal cortex (Valet et al., 2004), which can dampen nociception at the dorsal horn of the spine to reduce pain perception (Sprenger et al., 2012). Conversely, through connections with the amygdala and the insula, negative emotions can amplify pain perception (Wiech & Tracey, 2009) by increasing nociceptive activation in spinal neurons (Roy et al., 2009).

Central modulation of pain has been conserved across the 6 million years of human evolution by enhancing the survival value of our species. In situations of mortal threat (for our prehistoric ancestors, when being attacked by a saber-toothed tiger, or for modern humans, when marching into war), suppression of pain might enable a person who is severely injured to continue to flee from danger or successfully fight an otherwise deadly opponent. However, these same hardwired neurobiological circuits between the brain, the spinothalamic tract, the dorsal horn, and the peripheral nerves also provide a pathway by which negative emotions and stress can promote the amplification and chronification of pain, leading to impaired function and significant anguish.

Cognitive, Affective, Psychophysiological, and Behavioral Processes in Pain Perception and Regulation

In addition to the neurobiological circuits described above, pain also involves psychological processes, including attention to pain, pain appraisal, pain affect, and pain behavior. These processes are discussed below.

Attention to Pain: How Attention Affects Pain

Attention is the means by which certain pieces of information gain primacy over other pieces of information during the brain's competitive information processing (Desimone & Duncan, 1995). As a result, stimuli that are attended to receive preferential information processing and therefore become more likely to elicit behavioral responses. Pain automatically and involuntarily commands attention due to its relevance to bodily integrity and well-being (Eccleston & Crombez, 1999; Legrain et al., 2009). Yet, consciously regulating attention can also modify the perception of pain. Focusing attention on pain typically increases its perceived intensity (Quevedo & Coghill, 2007), whereas distracting attention from pain decreases its intensity (Terkelsen et al., 2004). That said, attention is a key facet of mindfulness, and MORE helps patients to cope with pain (see Chapter 3) by directing attention both toward ("zooming in") and away ("zooming out") from pain.

Redirecting attention away from pain changes pain-related activation in the brain. For instance, attentional distraction reduces pain-related activity in the somatosensory cortex, thalamus, and insula (Tracey & Mantyh, 2007). At the same time, distraction activates the prefrontal cortex, anterior cingulate cortex, and periaqueductal grey, suggesting that brain systems involved in attentional control of pain facilitate the descending pain modulatory system (Wiech et al., 2008). On the other hand, attentional hypervigilance for pain (Crombez et al., 2005)—that is, when people with chronic pain monitor and search their bodies for evidence of pain—magnifies pain intensity and is linked with interpreting harmless sensations (like tightness or tingling) as painfully unpleasant (Hollins et al., 2009; Rollman, 2009). When sustained over time, this maladaptive pattern of attention can result in a pain attentional bias, an automatic habit of paying attention to pain-related information at the exclusion of nonpainful sensations, objects, and events (Schoth et al., 2012).

Pain Appraisal: How Thoughts Affect Pain

The way we think about pain affects the way it is perceived. In other words, pain involves cognitive appraisal, whereby one consciously and unconsciously assesses the meaning of sensations to ascertain whether they signify present harm to the body or the potential threat of future harm. Pain appraisals are highly subjective—for example, professional bodybuilders or runners interpret the "burn" they feel in their muscles as pleasant and a sign of building muscle mass or stamina. Yet, someone new to exercise might view the same sensation as an indication of "overdoing it" and fear they have harmed themselves through exercise. The possibility of appraising the same stimulus as either harmful or not may stem from the dissociable neurobiological activity that mediates the sensory and emotional aspects of pain perception: Somatosensory cortex activity maps changes in pain intensity, whereas anterior cingulate cortex activity indexes changes in pain unpleasantness (Rainville et al., 1997, 1999). Consequently, two different people experiencing the same degree of pressure on their lumbar spine (as in during a massage) might perceive that sensation as either relaxing or agonizing, depending on how it is appraised. Thus, cognitive appraisal influences the perceived unpleasantness of pain (Price, 2002).

Pain appraisals not only involve an assessment of the threat value of a given sensation but also involve a determination of whether a person can cope with that sensation. If, during the cognitive appraisal process, available coping resources are deemed sufficient to manage the sensation, then pain may be perceived as controllable. When pain is perceived to be controllable, pain intensity is reduced via activation of the ventrolateral prefrontal cortex (Wiech et al., 2006; Woo et al., 2017). This same brain region is also involved in regulating negative emotions through reappraisal (Ochsner & Gross, 2005; Wager et al., 2008). Similarly, reinterpreting pain as a harmless sensation (e.g., warmth or tightness) leads to a greater sense of perceived control over pain (Haythornthwaite et al., 1998). Psychological interventions (like mindfulness) can reduce pain by teaching people to reinterpret pain sensations as harmless sensory information (e.g., sensations of warmth or tightness; Garland, Gaylord, et al., 2012). These findings directly inform the MORE treatment approach to dealing with pain. On the other hand, pain catastrophizing (i.e., viewing pain as unmanageable, ruminating about pain, and worrying that it will get worse or never go away) is associated with more pain intensity regardless of the degree of injury and physical impairment (Severeijns et al., 2001), and predicts the development of chronic pain (Edwards et al., 2016; Picavet et al., 2002) and poor outcomes following surgery (Dismore et al., 2020). People who have chronic pain may sometimes engage in pain catastrophizing, holding beliefs like "It's terrible and never going to get any better," "This pain means something serious is going to happen," and "I can't stand it anymore." These catastrophic ways of thinking can produce strong negative emotional reactions to pain.

Pain Affect: How Emotions Affect Pain

A person's emotional reaction to pain can also affect their perception of pain. Depending on how pain is cognitively appraised, it can lead to feelings of despair, fear, or anger. For instance, the belief "My pain is never going away; my future is hopeless," can lead to despair, whereas the belief "It's unjust that I have to live with chronic pain when other people live pain-free," is likely to lead to anger. Pain-related negative emotions co-occur with physiological reactions that amplify pain perception—for example, pain activates the sympathetic branch of the autonomic nervous system, marked by increased stress, muscle tension, fast heart rate, and exaggerated galvanic skin responses (Flor et al., 1985). Also, stress and negative emotions can activate skeletal muscle to produce painful muscle spasms (Lundberg et al., 1999), while increasing pain intensity and pain unpleasantness (Rainville et al., 2005). Although temporary and acute experiences of stress and negative emotions like fear and anger can dampen pain during the sympathetic "fight-or-flight" response through the release of norepinephrine (i.e., adrenaline), chronic activation of this response by stress can exacerbate the original injury by increasing blood flow and tension in injured muscle tissue (Cannon, 1929). Amplifying these autonomic effects, stress, catastrophizing, and negative emotional reactions to pain have endocrine and immune effects, including the release of proinflammatory cytokines and cortisol (Campbell et al., 2016; Edwards et al., 2008;

Quartana et al., 2010), that when sustained chronically increase nociception, delay healing, and aggravate tissue damage (Chapman et al., 2008; Sommer & Kress, 2004).

Furthermore, negative emotions activate the amygdala, anterior insula, and anterior cingulate cortex—brain structures that are also involved in turning attention toward pain and magnifying interoceptive awareness (i.e., the sense of the physical condition of the body; Craig, 2003; Wiech & Tracey, 2009). Consequently, when people feel afraid or angry due to pain or other stressors in their lives, activation in these brain regions boosts pain perception (de Wied & Verbaten, 2001; Kirwilliam & Derbyshire, 2008), increasing the likelihood that innocuous bodily sensations (e.g., pressure, tightness) will be interpreted as painful (Bogaerts et al., 2009; Panerai, 2011; Strigo et al., 2008). Relatedly, people with chronic pain often develop a fear of pain, manifested in hypervigilance and the tendency to scan the body for sensations of pain while avoiding movements that might induce pain (Keogh et al., 2001; Vlaeyen & Linton, 2012). Finally, negative emotions and stress can reduce the ability of the prefrontal cortex to regulate pain using cognitive coping strategies like reappraisal (Arnsten, 2009; Bushnell et al., 2013). Taken together, through this array of psychological, physiological, and neural processes, pain can lead to negative emotions that then amplify pain perception and the emotional anguish associated with pain.

Pain Behavior: How Behaviors Affect Pain

Finally, our behavioral reactions to pain can alleviate, sustain, or worsen pain experience. When people are in pain, they often exhibit pain behaviors like grimacing, rubbing, sighing, bracing, and guarding their movements (Keefe et al., 1984). These behaviors communicate when we are in pain and may elicit sympathy, acts of kindness, and lowered expectations from social relationships (Hadjistavropoulos et al., 2004). In this way, pain behaviors can reinforce pain experience. Similarly, muscular guarding and avoidance of physical activity may be negatively reinforced because these behaviors may temporarily alleviate pain (Turk & Flor, 1987). However, over time, activity avoidance may result in worse pain-related functional interference and disability (Buer & Linton, 2002; Klenerman et al., 1995; Linton et al., 2000). People with chronic pain often develop these maladaptive pain behaviors, which then become entrenched through the reinforcement processes described above. Alternatively, gradual, incremental increases in physical activity and exercise in spite of pain have been shown to reduce pain intensity, disability, physical impairment, and psychological distress for people with chronic pain (Geneen et al., 2017).

Chronic Pain by "Default": A Role for Default Mode Networks in the Development of a Pain-Related Identity

As pain becomes chronic, its progression is associated with the interaction among original injury, changes in the nervous system, and cognitive-affective dysregulation (Apkarian et al., 2005; Borsook et al., 2018; Hashmi et al., 2013). The experience of pain may become less of a direct "readout" of nociceptive signals from the injury, and more of a pattern in the brain that encodes particular habits of attention, emotion, thought, and memory. Inferences and predictions derived from past pain episodes may result in biased interpretations of the body's current state that accumulate into cognitive schemas that preserve and exacerbate pain—that is, rather than actually sensing the current physiological condition of the body, a person with chronic pain might experience the painful sensations they expect or believe they will experience. For instance, patients who live with pain for many years come to expect they will feel pain in the future, thinking, "My pain is never going to go away—my life is over," and this expectation can become a self-fulfilling prophecy. Indeed, there is evidence that the brain constructs pain from these sorts of expectations (Wiech, 2016) by increasing the likelihood that innocuous sensations will be interpreted as painful. As such, self-referential thought processes appear to play a role in chronic pain. Self-referential thought (i.e., thinking about yourself or your own life story) is reflected by oscillating activity in a network of brain regions that are activated when we are at rest and allowing our minds to wander (posterior cingulate cortex/precuneus, medial prefrontal cortex, and the inferior and lateral temporal cortices), referred to as the default mode network (DMN; Raichle et al., 2001). People with chronic pain have abnormal DMN activity and altered connections between the DMN and brain regions that mediate sensory processing (Alshelh et al., 2018; Baliki et al., 2008, 2014; Loggia et al., 2013; Wasan et al., 2011). Hypothetically, dysregulation of DMN activity may cause pain to become the primary object of self-referential processing (Zeidan & Coghill, 2013), whereby one's sense of identity and life story become entrapped and dominated by pain-related memories and associations. From a clinical perspective, if one says, "I am in pain" enough times, the preposition "in" eventually gets dropped, and "I am in pain" becomes "I am pain" as the sense of self becomes largely identified with chronic pain. When one's identity becomes fused with the experience of chronic pain, pain attentional biases predominate, leading a person to notice only the physically and emotionally painful moments in their life, and therefore they see no possibility of change, no hope for the future.

> A person's sense of identity can become dominated by pain-related memories and associations.

The Downward Spiral from Chronic Pain to Opioid Misuse and OUD

To alleviate pain and pain-related emotional suffering, many patients and their physicians turn to opioid medications. These powerful medications interact with endogenous opioid systems in the brain. Both exogenous opioids (e.g., opioid medications) and endogenous opioids (those naturally produced by the body, such as beta-endorphin and enkephalins) activate *mu*, *kappa*, and *delta* opioid receptors throughout multiple regions across the brain, including the cerebral cortex, periaqueductal grey, thalamus, hypothalamus, and spinal cord, among other structures (Arvidsson et al., 1995; Lewis et al., 1983; Mathieu-Kia et al., 2001; Pan & Pasternak, 2011; Traynor & Wood, 1987). The activation of mu opioid receptors results in the analgesic effects of opioid drugs (Fields, 2011; Julien, 2007). However, mu receptor agonists (i.e., drugs that activate mu opioid receptors, such as those listed above) also indirectly excite dopamine-secreting neurons in the ventral tegmental area (Chiara & North, 1992; Johnson & North, 1992) and modulate reward processing in the brain (Meier et al., 2021). The effect of opioids on dopamine neurotransmission appears to be a key component of the reinforcing and rewarding properties of opioids, and therefore is integral to the development and maintenance of opioid addiction (Berridge et al., 2009; Le Merrer et al., 2009; Volkow et al., 2011).

Effects of Opioids on the Brain

When a person who has never taken opioids is administered a drug like morphine, brain regions involved in reward processing including the nucleus accumbens, the amygdala, and the orbitofrontal cortex become activated (Becerra et al., 2006; Leppä et al., 2006; Wanigasekera et al., 2012), which together produce the euphoria and pleasure of the opioid "high." At the same time, brain regions involved in cognitive control and attention become deactivated (e.g., dorsolateral prefrontal cortex, anterior cingulate cortex, inferior parietal lobe; Becerra et al., 2006; Jastrzab et al., 2012; Lee et al., 2014). In that regard, multiple studies have shown that opioids cause cognitive impairments (Baldacchino et al., 2012; Zacny, 1995). As the opioid dose is increased, neural activity in the brain stem and medial thalamus are decreased, resulting in sedation and diminished functioning to the point of unconsciousness (Becerra et al., 2006), ultimately leading to the fatal cessation of breathing during overdoses. Plausibly, when people who are at high risk for developing addiction are first exposed to opioids, they may experience a strong activation of their brain's reward circuitry coupled with decreased activation in brain regions involved in self-control, a pattern of brain activation that makes it difficult for them to stop using opioids. Opioid-induced deficits in executive function, compounded with those associated with chronic pain (Berryman et al., 2014), may undermine a patient's ability to use cognitive coping strategies to manage pain without drugs, leading to increased dependence on opioids for pain relief.

The Neurobiological Progression from Opioid Dependence to Opioid Attentional Bias and Hedonic Dysregulation

LTOT for chronic pain puts vulnerable people at risk for engaging in opioid misuse and potentially even developing OUD. When medically appropriate opioid use is sustained over weeks and months, physical dependence symptoms can emerge as a result of changes in the brain that cause tolerance (i.e., needing higher doses of opioids to achieve the same effect), withdrawal (i.e., unpleasant symptoms when opioids are discontinued), and, in some cases, opioid-induced hyperalgesia (Chu et al., 2008): an increased sensitivity to pain. These physical symptoms of opioid dependence do not necessarily signify OUD and instead simply reflect the pharmacological effects of LTOT on the brain. In contrast, the loss of control over opioid use that is characteristic of addiction occurs when reward learning mechanisms become hijacked

> Even medically appropriate opioid use can lead to dependence and other problems.

by repeated opioid use, resulting in durable changes to brain structure and function of the brain (known as *neuroplasticity*) as compulsive, addictive habits are formed (Everitt & Robbins, 2016; Kalivas & O'Brien, 2008).

The path from medically appropriate opioid use to OUD involves progressive dysregulation of dopamine-rich areas of the brain, including the orbitofrontal cortex, ventral tegmental area, and the ventral striatum that are central to the reward learning process (Koob & Volkow, 2016). When opioids result in pain relief or euphoria, conditioned stimuli associated with opioid use are imbued with value and become more salient through these dopamine circuits (Berridge & Robinson, 2016; Robinson & Berridge, 2000). Thus, the brain comes to learn to seek opioids and focus on opioid-related cues (e.g., an opioid pill bottle, a prescription slip, or an advertisement from the pharmacy where opioids are dispensed) as a means of maintaining a sense of well-being. Opioid cues may become salient through the reward, pleasure, and euphoria produced by opioid use (positive reinforcement) or through the effects of opioids on reducing physical or emotional pain (negative reinforcement; Fields, 2004). Such reward learning can lead to a strong motivation to take opioids (a "wanting" for opioids, also known as opioid *craving*), even in the absence of consciously preferring or enjoying the drug (a "liking" for opioids; Berridge & Robinson, 2016; Robinson & Berridge, 2000). In that regard, many people with chronic pain report disliking opioids because of their side effects (e.g., drowsiness, nausea) and/or the stigma associated with opioid use, yet they nevertheless may feel a strong, compulsive wanting or craving to take opioids just to feel okay.

With chronic use of opioids over months and years, the temporary brain changes produced by opioids become more stable as the person begins to form the automatic habit of opioid use (i.e., automaticity; see Chapter 1), mediated by structural and functional changes in deep brain structures, like the hippocampus, amygdala, and striatum (Yin & Knowlton, 2006). Recurrent drug use is believed to lead to the development of automatic drug use action schemas—that is, memory patterns that unconsciously govern and coordinate consumption of the drug through automatized sequences of behavior (Everitt & Robbins, 2016; Piazza & Deroche-Gamonet, 2013; Tiffany, 1990). In other words, drug use can become an automatic habit that can develop a life of its own; as the old proverb goes, "First the man takes a drink, then the drink takes a drink, and finally the drink takes the man." Opioid use can operate on "autopilot," in much the same way as other complex thought–action repertoires can be engaged without conscious volition by conditioned contextual cues (Chartrand & Bargh, 1999), like the commonplace occurrence of driving without being fully conscious of the road, the route, or the turns you took to get to your destination. Automatic drug use schema may arise out of a history of repeated drug use in much the same way that other overlearned behavioral repertoires become automatized (e.g., riding a bike, driving a car). Stimulus–response habits are established through repetition and reinforcement. After hundreds of repetitions of consistent responses to a given stimulus, attending and responding to that stimulus become automatic (Shiffrin & Schneider, 1977). During the formation of automatic habits, a neurobiological shift occurs in which behaviors that were originally guided by thoughtful expectation and prediction of potential outcomes become controlled by sensorimotor cortico-basal ganglia networks (Yin & Knowlton, 2006).

As a result of the development of the opioid use habit, cues associated with past opioid use are able to automatically capture attention—for example, imagine a man who is in between opioid doses, who has been waiting for nearly 4 hours to take his next dose, but still has to wait another 20 minutes before dosing. He is in the bathroom, brushing his teeth, and above the sink is a medicine cabinet, where his oxycodone bottle is stored. What do you think he is thinking about in that moment? And even if this man would rather be focusing elsewhere, he may find his attention drawn back and back again to the pills that are 6 inches from his face. This phenomenon, known as addiction attentional bias (Field & Cox, 2008), is similar to the pain attentional bias previously discussed, and can cause craving (Field et al., 2009), irrespective of the need for pain relief. Although addiction attentional bias has been most often observed in people who develop substance use disorders for illicit drugs, my own laboratory was the first to demonstrate the presence of an opioid attentional bias among people with chronic pain with OUD (Garland, Froeliger, Passik, et al., 2013). We later found that patients with the strongest attentional bias toward opioids were the most likely to misuse opioids 20 weeks following the end of treatment (Garland & Howard, 2014), suggesting that opioid attentional bias has important clinical consequences.

Through conditioning processes, pain also becomes associated with the opioid use habit. When a person with chronic pain experiences relief after initiating opioid use, the experience of pain eventually comes to serve as a conditioned stimulus that elicits the conditioned response of opioid use. Because opioids target brain regions rich in opioid receptors that are involved in processing negative emotions (e.g., the amygdala), opioids can relieve emotional pain perhaps even more potently than physical pain (Ballantyne & Sullivan, 2017; Koob, 2020). Many people with long-standing depression, anxiety, or PTSD report that the first time they tried opioids was the first time in their entire lives when they felt completely at peace. As such, some people with chronic pain on LTOT take opioids to alleviate sadness, fear, anger, and stress, in addition to their physical pain. This kind of opioid misuse is seductive in that it temporarily works to reduce distress, and through the process of negative reinforcement conditioning (Carpenter, Lane, et al., 2019) strengthens the opioid use habit. It is for this reason that people with high levels of negative affect, psychiatric disorders, and trauma histories are more likely to misuse opioids (Ives et al., 2006; Martel et al., 2014; Sullivan et al., 2010).

When paired with the experience of elevated pain (whether physical or emotional), opioid cues may produce an especially potent conditioned drug-seeking response. In the typical associative learning sequence, pain precedes opioid use and thus may prime the opioid use habit when followed by opioid cues (Garland, Bryan, et al., 2018). However, when people begin to misuse opioids for the euphoria they can produce, this associative learning process may evolve such that opioid cues trigger opioid use, whether or not pain is present. Thus, as a patient with chronic pain who misuses opioids progresses toward opioid addiction, the normative associative learning process that had paired pain and opioid use becomes dysregulated such that the motivation to seek opioids is largely decoupled from pain and driven by opioid cues that have acquired incentive salience through habit learning. Because opioid use activates mesolimbic dopamine during the experience of reward (i.e., the opioid high or the relief of physical or emotional pain), this leads to a strengthening of synaptic connections in neural pathways that govern the opioid-seeking behavior associated with that reward. Consequently, when external (e.g., the sight of a pill bottle) or internal (e.g., pain, stress) cues associated with past opioid use capture attention, they trigger a similar pattern of dopamine release that activates the opioid use habit (Pantazis et al., 2021).

In addition to increasing sensitivity to opioid-related cues, chronic opioid use and misuse may decrease sensitivity of brain reward circuits (orbitofrontal cortex, ventral striatum) to natural, non-drug rewards like food, sex, and social connections (Ballantyne & Sullivan, 2017; Bommersbach et al., 2020; Koob, 2020; Volkow et al., 2019). As the brain becomes more sensitive to opioid-related cues over time, the reward value of opioids comes to outweigh the reward derived from naturally rewarding objects and events in the social environment (e.g., a beautiful sunset, a smiling baby, a cuddly puppy, the caress of a loved one, or the sense of a job well-done). When opioids usurp the reward value of people, places, and things that the person once felt were meaningful, OUD takes hold, and seeking and taking opioids become more important than anything else in life. Reduced responsiveness to natural rewards relative to drug-related cues can be seen in the brains of people addicted to heroin using EEG (Lubman et al., 2008) and MRI (Huang et al., 2024). This reduced neurophysiological response to images representing natural rewards relative to heroin images significantly predicts future opiate use (Lubman et al., 2009). People with chronic pain who misuse and are addicted to prescription opioids also exhibit blunting of responses to natural rewards (Garland, Bryan, et al., 2017; Garland, Froeliger, et al., 2015a; Garland, Trøstheim, et al., 2020; Huhn et al., 2021), and a blunted natural reward response is associated with heightened opioid craving (Garland, Bryan, et al., 2017; Huang et al., 2024). This neurophysiological insensitivity to natural reward may underpin *anhedonia*—the reduced ability to experience pleasure—which has been shown to be elevated in people with OUD and those with chronic pain who misuse opioids (Garfield et al., 2014; Garland, Trøstheim, et al., 2020). As a result of these changes in brain reward circuitry, eventually a patient who repeatedly misuses opioids may become less able to feel a sense of pleasure, joy, and meaning from everyday life, creating an empty hole that pushes them to take higher and higher doses of opioids to preserve a dwindling sense of well-being.

At the same time, chronic opioid use and misuse can cause neuroplastic changes to the extended amygdala, increasing the sensitivity of the individual to emotional distress (Koob, 2020). Consequently, people with chronic pain who misuse opioids may develop hyperkatifeia: a negative emotional state that drives them to continue to take escalating doses of opioids to alleviate the powerful feelings of malaise, irritability, anxiety, and dysphoria that occur each time the drug wears off (Shurman et al., 2010). Compounding this problem, my own studies have shown that opioid misuse is associated with an inability to regulate negative emotions through reappraisal (Garland, Bryan, et al., 2017; Garland, Hanley, et al., 2018; Garland, Reese, et al., 2019; Hudak et al., 2022). Instead of reappraisal, people may try to suppress negative emotions, which eventually backfires (Wegner, 1994) and increases opioid craving (Garland, Brown, et al., 2016). Through all of the aforementioned changes to stress and reward circuitry in the brain, repeated opioid misuse leads to *hedonic dysregulation*, a disruption of the basic balance of well-being characterized by hyperalgesia, anhedonia, and hyperkatifeia, ensnaring the individual in a vicious cycle where the perceived solution (i.e., opioid use) to their problem (i.e., pain and distress) only magnifies the problem.

Finally, like chronic pain, addiction involves aberrant default-mode self-referential processing (Zhang & Volkow, 2019). Repeated rumination on addiction-related thoughts and cravings day after day may result in addiction becoming entrenched in the sense of self. During this process, the drug gains primary self-relevance, and it becomes a central point of meaning in life at the expense of nondrug natural rewards. One's identity becomes fused with addiction and embedded into the default mode of the self.

Taken together, the downward spiral linking chronic pain to opioid misuse and OUD involves a cycle of behavioral escalation, in which physical pain, cognitive biases, and emotional suffering interact to drive a person to take increasingly higher doses of opioids in an attempt to preserve a dwindling sense of hedonic well-being. This vain attempt comes at an ironic and serious cost, altering stress and reward thresholds in the brain that render the individual more sensitive to physical and emotional pain, more captivated by opioid-related cues and craving, and less responsive to natural, healthy rewards—a vicious cycle that propels opioid misuse toward full-blown addictive behavior. Eventually, this path may lead to the loss of control over opioid use that is characteristic of OUD. This downward spiral is why I believe the term *disease of despair* is not a mere metaphor but is instead an apt description of the underlying factors that drive an opioid crisis. In the next chapter, I discuss how to treat the disease of despair and interrupt the downward spiral by stimulating an upward spiral from mindfulness to meaning.

Chapter 3

What Is MORE and How Can It Help?

Because pain, maladaptive cognitions, negative emotions, automaticity, attentional biases, and hedonic dysregulation propel the downward spiral, therapies that address these mechanisms can strengthen the recovery process. To that end, MORE was specifically designed to target each of these mechanisms with evidence-based techniques and principles drawn from mindfulness training, "third-wave" CBT, and positive psychology. From these three great psychotherapeutic traditions, MORE's efficacy rests on three corresponding pillars: mindfulness, reappraisal, and savoring. In turn, these pillars are thought to support the emergence of a fourth therapeutic process—*self-transcendence*—the sense of being connected to something greater than the self.

Mindfulness

Mindfulness is the foundation of MORE. Every MORE session includes mindfulness techniques. Given the centrality of mindfulness to MORE, this concept deserves a detailed discussion. Mindfulness training is the foundational contemplative practice of ancient Indo–Sino–Tibetan traditions. Following the migration of mindfulness into the West around the beginning of the 20th century, it began to spread in the 1960s and 1970s as a spiritual practice before being translated into health care through the seminal Mindfulness-Based Stress Reduction (MBSR) program pioneered by Jon Kabat-Zinn (1982, 1990, 2011, 2019), who was arguably the first to successfully bring mindfulness to mainstream medicine. Early research on MBSR and its neurobiological mechanisms (e.g., Davidson et al., 2003) led to the birth of an entire scientific field, known as contemplative science, dedicated to understanding the nature of mindfulness and how it could be applied to enhance human health. The flowering of contemplative science resulted in a meteoric rise in the number of research studies and scientific articles on mindfulness. To date, over 16,000 papers on mindfulness have been published in academic journals (Baminiwatta & Solangaarachchi, 2021), and as of 2022, the National Institutes of Health (NIH) are currently funding more than $146 million in active grants on mindfulness. As a result, mindfulness has made a massive contribution to science and health care.

Numerous modern conceptualizations of mindfulness have been put forth by scientists and clinicians in fields like medicine and psychology, based on reinterpretations of teachings from Theravada, Mahayana, Zen (or Ch'an), and Vajrayana Buddhist traditions. These schools of Buddhism have strongly influenced American and European culture, and therefore have come to dominate Western conceptual frameworks of mindfulness. Yet, other Asian philosophies, including Advaita Vedanta, Taoism, and the Nondual Tantra of Kashmir Shaivism also have much to offer in elucidating this construct, and each has influenced MORE in kind. Regardless of its ancient spiritual roots, in the West mindfulness is now a secular concept, stripped of its religious content, and defined in terms of its neurocognitive mechanisms.

In the modern scientific literature, mindfulness is often operationalized and measured as a state, trait, and practice. The *state of mindfulness* has been characterized by a nonreactive meta-awareness and acceptance of moment-by-moment thoughts, emotions, perceptions, and sensations without fixation on thoughts of past and future (Lutz et al., 2008; Vago & Silbersweig, 2012). Although the term *state* implies a somewhat static entity, the state of mindfulness is anything but static. Others have termed mindfulness a "process" to capture the dynamical action of mindfulness (Bishop et al., 2004; Teasdale, 2022). From a cognitive science perspective, mindfulness is an emergent property of consciousness arising out of the interaction of multiple mental mechanisms (e.g., attention regulation, working memory, inhibitory control, and meta-awareness), propelled by dynamical activations of multiple neural networks working in concert across the brain.

Among such cognitive mechanisms, in my view, the construct of meta-awareness is integral to the therapeutic power of mindfulness. At any moment, human consciousness can operate on two levels: the *object* level of awareness and the *meta*-level of awareness. The object level of awareness consists of the contents of our mind (e.g., thoughts, emotions, body sensations) that we pay attention to as they flit in and out of the field of awareness. In contrast, the meta-level of awareness monitors the content of consciousness (the object level) while having the capacity to reflect back upon the process of consciousness itself without being anchored to a particular object (Dunne et al., 2019; Nelson et al., 1999). In other words, in addition to being aware of mental objects (e.g., a thought, an itch on my left leg), I can also become aware of the quality of my awareness (e.g., "Am I sleepy?"; "Is my mind clear?"; "Is my mind quiet?"; "Am I paying attention?"). Meta-awareness is this self-reflexive aspect of the mind—the awareness of awareness—that extends beyond any particular mental content. Meta-awareness allows one to decenter from the objects of awareness (e.g., a painful body sensation, emotion, or thought)—that is, rather than being "wrapped up" and immersed in a thought or feeling, we can attain psychological distance from those mental objects by translocating the center of awareness beyond the object to the field in which they arise (e.g., "My leg itches, but does the field of awareness in which the itch occurs itch?"). Through *decentering* (another key component of mindfulness), we come to view those objects as transitory mental events, lacking inherent truth or permanence. Through meta-awareness "one realizes 'this pain is not me,' 'this depression is not me,' 'these thoughts are not me'" (Shapiro et al., 2006, p. 378). In other words, one becomes like a witness to the arising, sustenance, and ceasing of mental contents. However, with this explanation I do not intend to reify "the witness" or imply that the meta-awareness evoked by mindfulness creates some duality between observer and observed. To avoid such dualisms, it may be more apt to simply state that mindfulness involves the process of witnessing experience unfold in the field of awareness.

In some traditions (e.g., Kashmir Shavisim), the practice of mindfulness is thought to lead to this witness consciousness (*turiya*), a "fourth state" beyond waking, dreaming, and deep sleep (Wallis, 2017). The practice of inverting awareness upon itself can deepen to a point in which the objects of awareness are transcended; as the salience of mental objects begins to fade, the space of awareness that surrounds and holds the object comes into focus. Resting the focus of the mind in spacious awareness beyond mental objects is accompanied by a quieting of self-referential thought. From the perspective of meta-awareness, thoughts are held to "self-liberate"—they become transparent, effervescent, transitory, and unreal, like a mist, cloud, bubble, mirage, or daydream. As thoughts recede, the resultant mental quiescence can paradoxically be both empty of content and full of wakefulness, and has been characterized as an empty luminous cognizance in the Mahāmudrā tradition of Buddhism. When it reaches its zenith, meta-awareness can mature into a form of *nondual awareness*, a state of pure consciousness that is largely (or completely) devoid of the subject–object duality that structures normal human consciousness (Josipovic, 2014; Metzinger, 2024). "Nondual awareness that transcends intellect is nonconceptual, lucid, like all-pervading space. . . . It is lucid and indefinable, without center or circumference, unstained, undefiled, and free from fear and desire" (Namgyal, 2006, p. 94). The self-transcendent state of pure consciousness or nondual awareness is often characterized by a fading of the sense of self or a sense of oneness, coupled with expansive positive emotional qualities, ranging from peace to joy, love, or even ecstatic bliss (Hanley et al., 2018; Metzinger, 2024). The concept of self-transcendence is discussed in detail in Chapter 7.

The *practice of mindfulness* consists of meditation techniques designed to cultivate the state of mindfulness. Mindfulness meditation practice involves repeatedly focusing attention on an object while monitoring the field of awareness and alternately acknowledging and letting go of distracting thoughts and emotions by reorienting attention back to the object. Objects of mindfulness practice can include the sensation of the breath; sensations in the body; visual stimuli, such as the expanse of a clear sky or a body of water, like a stream or ocean; mental contents, such as thoughts or feelings; or the field of awareness itself (Dunne et al., 2019; Namgyal, 2006). MORE includes training in all of these forms of mindfulness practice.

Finally, the *trait of mindfulness* has been defined as the dispositional propensity toward exhibiting nonjudgmental, nonreactive awareness of one's thoughts, emotions, experiences, and actions in everyday life, even when not engaged in mindfulness meditation (Baer et al., 2006). Research indicates that people vary in the extent to which they exhibit trait mindfulness, yet this dispositionality can be strengthened through training. Mindful people tend to have better physical and mental health, whereas people who tend toward mindlessness (i.e., absent-mindedly falling into self-destructive habits) are less healthy and suffer from more severe addictive behaviors (Carpenter, Conroy, et al., 2019; Karyadi et al., 2014; Sala et al., 2020), including opioid misuse (Priddy et al., 2018). Indeed, people who participate in MBIs like MORE evidence increases in trait mindfulness, which mediates the effects of training on clinical outcomes (Gu et al., 2015). This discovery can bring hope, suggesting that even if someone begins MORE with a low level of trait mindfulness, they can make themselves into a more mindful person with dedicated practice.

It may be fruitful to conceptualize mindfulness as a *state-by-trait interaction*—that is, each time you activate the state of mindfulness by practicing mindfulness meditation, this leaves lasting traces in the mind (and brain) that can accrue into durable changes in trait mindfulness (Garland, Fredrickson, et al., 2010; Goleman & Davidson, 2018), possibly mediated through neuroplasticity and experience-dependent alterations in gene expression (Black et al., 2019; Garland & Howard, 2009). Indeed, my own research has shown that increases in the trajectory of state mindfulness from one meditation practice session to another lead to the development of greater trait mindfulness (Kiken et al., 2015). And, some studies (though not all; see Kral et al., 2022) suggest that mindfulness practice can lead to durable structural changes in parts of the brain that subserve emotion regulation, learning, memory, and the ability to shift one's perspective (Fox et al., 2014; Holzel et al., 2011; R. Tang et al., 2020; Y.-Y. Tang et al., 2010, 2012; Valk et al., 2017). In other words, mindfulness can be used to change not only the function but possibly even the structure of the brain.

That said, we should consider the scientific operationalization of mindfulness as a state and trait as "convenient designations" or ways of describing the data rather than ontological truths. In truth there is no one mindful state. Mindfulness involves meta-awareness and acceptance of whatever arises in the mind in any moment. For instance, if one cultivates meta-awareness and acceptance of feelings of calm and relaxation, that is mindfulness. If one cultivates meta-awareness and acceptance of feelings of pain or craving, that is mindfulness. If one cultivates meta-awareness and acceptance of worries and regrets, that is mindfulness. In this sense, mindfulness may be construed as the ensemble of all possible states (Jon Kabat-Zinn, personal communication, February 5, 2024). One of the key dangers of defining mindfulness as a particular state and trait is that it may reify the image of an idealized better place or mental quality as the goal. This reification may then in turn foster seeking or craving on the part of the practitioner to "obtain" or "achieve" this better place or mental quality, thereby rejecting what is actually present in the moment. This attitude is the antithesis of mindfulness. Instead, mindfulness shows us that awareness is larger than and can hold even difficult mind states, and thus is intrinsically free and already whole.

Reappraisal

Reappraisal is both a stress-coping process that people naturally engage in and the cornerstone of CBT, an evidence-based treatment approach that has been studied and used since the 1970s. As a means of coping, reappraisal is the process of reframing the meaning of an adverse life event so as to see that event as more benign, or even as a potential source of benefit or psychological growth (Lazarus & Folkman, 1984). When one appraises a given life situation as a potential threat or present harm, and believes they are unable to successfully resolve the situation, stress arises. This initial appraisal process can be automatic, executed without conscious deliberation (Chartrand & Bargh, 1999), and is mediated by limbic structures in the brain like the amygdala, which rapidly process stimuli for their threat value (LeDoux, 2003). However, conscious reflection on the meaning of the stimulus and its situational context, as well as one's own strengths, capabilities, and resources, can lead to a reinterpretation of the stressor as being less adverse than initially appraised, or potentially, even a means of learning or growing as a person (e.g., "Facing this situation has made me a stronger person"). In other words, through reappraisal one's mental model of the stressor and its context is transformed (Teasdale, 2022). This slower, deliberate process of cognitive reappraisal has been shown to regulate negative emotions by increasing prefrontal cortical control over activity in the amygdala (Ochsner & Gross, 2005; Wager et al., 2008) and to activate nodes of the corticostriatal reward circuit integral to the attribution of positive meaning, including ventral striatum and medial prefrontal cortex (Doré et al., 2017).

Reappraisal is also an empirically supported CBT technique, known as *cognitive restructuring* (i.e., the process of identifying and modifying maladaptive thoughts via methods such as logical disputation). Many hundreds of well-controlled research studies have shown that CBT is an effective means of treating a wide range of conditions, with meta-analyses showing that CBT is significantly more effective than other psychotherapies at treating emotional problems (e.g., Tolin, 2010). MORE provides instruction in "mindful reappraisal" by using mindfulness to facilitate the process of reappraisal (Garland et al., 2009). Indeed, well-controlled experimental research demonstrates that the process of decentering inherent in mindfulness promotes reappraisal (Wang et al., 2023), and observational studies indicate that mindfulness practice and reappraisal mutually facilitate each other with the dynamics of an upward spiral (Garland, Kiken, et al., 2017). Mindfulness facilitates reappraisal in that "the central process in mindfulness is the flexible creation of novel, tailor-made, mental models of experience (or the fine-tuning of existing mental models), moment after moment after moment" (Teasdale, 2022, p. 97). Moreover, the positive mental states generated by mindfulness practice turn attention toward what is beautiful, rewarding, or meaningful in life and thereby strengthen positive interpretations of the current situation (Garland, Farb, et al., 2015a). As people become more mindful, they tend to reappraise the stressors in their lives as opportunities for personal growth, which accounts for some of the stress-reductive effects of mindfulness (Garland, Gaylord, et al., 2011). This process of mindful reappraisal may involve activation of the medial, ventrolateral, and dorsolateral prefrontal cortices—and indeed, neuroimaging research shows that mindfulness training augments activity in these brain regions during reappraisal (Goldin et al., 2021).

> Mindful reappraisal can help regulate negative emotions.

Savoring

Savoring is a core construct from positive psychology, the scientific study of characteristics, virtues, and strengths that allows individuals to flourish (Seligman et al., 2006). Savoring involves attending to the pleasant sensory features (e.g., visual, auditory, gustatory, olfactory, tactile, or kinesthetic) of a naturally rewarding stimulus while turning meta-awareness toward the positive emotions and pleasurable sensations that emerge during contact with the stimulus (Bryant & Veroff, 2017). In this sense, savoring involves an aspect of mindfulness. Insofar as mindfulness can sharpen sensory perception unclouded by emotional biases and preconceived notions, allowing us to view the present moment with a heightened degree of "freshness," mindfulness has been shown to amplify brain markers of attention to positive emotional stimuli (Egan et al., 2017). Consequently, mindfulness may increase reward experience from naturally rewarding objects and events (Arch et al., 2016; Geschwind et al., 2011). Mindfulness promotes the savoring of natural rewards by stabilizing and reorienting attention from distraction onto the pleasant stimulus, and then by deepening meta-awareness of positive emotional and interoceptive responses to the stimulus (Garland, Farb, et al., 2015a).

MORE leverages this synergy via a mindful savoring technique in which patients are first taught to attend to the pleasant colors, textures, and scents of a rose, as well as the touch of its petals against the skin, while remaining sensitive to their own emotional response to the flower (see Session 4). As patients become aware of pleasurable sensations or positive emotions, they are then instructed to turn their attention inward, and mindfully savor the pleasant feelings arising in their mind or body, as well as any emotional associations or meaningful insights that occur during the savoring practice. When the pleasant sensations and positive emotions begin to fade, patients are encouraged to shift their attention outward again to appreciate the flower once more. This toggling of exteroceptive and interoceptive attention on a wide variety of pleasant perceptions, sensations, cognitions, emotions, and memories might overcome the "hedonic treadmill effect" (Brickman & Campbell, 1971) that causes people to quickly adapt to and thereby lose pleasure from a positive stimulus. After learning this technique, in Session 4, patients in MORE are instructed to practice mindful savoring with other, more personally meaningful pleasant objects and events that naturally occur in their everyday lives, as a means of coping with difficult experience and amplifying positive emotions.

In the same way that we can analogize mindfulness meditation as a form of exercise or a workout for the prefrontal cortex, savoring might be construed as a means of exercising the key nodes of the brain's reward circuit, including the orbitofrontal cortex and ventral striatum. Such exercise is particularly important, given the tendency in modern society for individuals to continually seek more and more intense forms of stimulation in the pursuit of pleasure. This pursuit of pleasure might be likened to an addiction. And, as in addiction, the phenomenon of tolerance can occur. We seek richer and tastier foods, fancier clothes and bigger houses, more stimulating company, increasingly exciting and exotic vacations, and a growing number of likes and followers on social media to preserve an ever-dwindling sense of happiness. Due to allostatic processes in the brain, the reward system may become "flabby," and require a more intense stimulus to elicit a smaller sense of reward. Savoring might reverse this process, by increasing sensitivity to more and more subtle everyday pleasures. By strengthening the tone of the reward system through the exercise of savoring, an apparently mildly pleasurable stimulus like the coolness of a breeze, a birdsong, a stranger's smile, a flower growing in a sidewalk crack, or even the sense of one's body resting in a chair may become sources of delight and wonder.

In that regard, across multiple studies, MORE has been shown to increase subjective, autonomic, and neurophysiological responses during the savoring of natural rewards in people suffering from chronic pain and opioid misuse (Garland et al., 2014, 2023; Garland, Atchley, et al., 2019), nicotine addiction (Froeliger et al., 2017), and obesity (Thomas et al., 2019). And, across these studies, increases in natural reward processing were associated with reductions in craving, substance use or misuse, and attentional bias, providing robust support for the restructuring reward hypothesis (see Chapter 1 and the section "MORE Aims to Restructure Reward Processing," below). Savoring also decreases pain by activating reward circuitry in the brain (Finan et al., 2022).

> Savoring boosts positive emotions and amplifies healthy pleasure.

Mindfulness, reappraisal, and savoring are the three pillars of MORE. Yet, there is a fourth dimension of MORE, an emergent property that arises out of the practice of these three skills: self-transcendence. *Self-transcendence* is the profound sense of interconnectedness with something greater than the self (Yaden et al., 2017). During self-transcendent experience, the sense of one's self as an isolated being, encapsulated and delimited by the skin, can temporarily fade, revealing an experiential unity between the self and the world, a form of *nondual awareness* in which subject and object are unified. This sense of oneness is pregnant with meaning and motivates prosocial acts of compassion and empathy. Indeed, meaning making may reach its apex in self-transcendence, which was classically held to be the *sine qua non* of addiction recovery (e.g., surrendering to a higher power in Alcoholics Anonymous [AA]) and integral to disrupting the maladaptive cognitive patterns that fuel addiction (Bateson, 1971). Though self-transcendence can arise spontaneously during awe and other naturally occurring peak experiences, it may also be engendered by mindfulness meditation and other contemplative practices (Hanley et al., 2018; Wahbeh et al., 2018) whose original soteriological purpose was to foster states in which the subject–object dichotomy that structures ordinary human consciousness is transcended by the experience of a nondual awareness as described above (Josipovic, 2014).

Drawing on techniques, skills, and principles derived from mindfulness training, CBT, and positive psychology, MORE is a targeted intervention that aims to ameliorate addiction, emotional distress, and chronic pain through a number of specific therapeutic mechanisms detailed in the section "The Therapeutic Mechanisms of MORE," below. Here I offer theoretical rationale and research evidence in support of these hypothetical mechanisms of action.

The Mindfulness-to-Meaning Theory

MORE is grounded in the mindfulness-to-meaning theory (MMT; Garland, Farb, et al., 2015a) a temporally dynamic process model of mindful positive emotion regulation that elucidates the downstream cognitive-affective mechanisms by which mindfulness promotes human flourishing (see Figure 3.1). The MMT proposes that mindfulness facilitates decentering from stressors (like chronic pain and addiction) into a state of meta-awareness that disrupts negative attentional biases and maladaptive cognitive schemas, and broadens attention to encompass an enlarged set of contextual data from which new, adaptive appraisals of self and world can be constructed. Integrating this widened array of positive, neutral, and negative contextual features within the broadened scope of awareness facilitates reappraisal of adversity as a source of psychological growth. In turn, the positive emotions stimulated by this mindful reappraisal process can be further amplified through the use of mindfulness to savor the hedonic features and higher-order affective meaning of the situational context—propelling an upward spiral of positive affect and cognition toward a sense of meaning in life, and leading to self-transcendence, the sense of being connected to something greater than the self. Ultimately, this salutogenic upward spiral may reach its apex in nondual awareness (Garland & Fredrickson, 2019).

Given the MMT as a foundation, self-transcendence naturally emerges out of the interaction of mindfulness, reappraisal, and savoring skills taught in MORE, but is also directly pointed to in the MORE meditation practices, the MORE processing approach, and in the psychoeducational material. This direct pointing is aligned with "pointing out instructions" in the Mahāmudrā (Namgyal, 2006) and Dzogchen traditions (Rinpoche, 2013) of Tibetan Buddhism designed to rapidly awaken the meditation practitioner to the realization that all "appearances are mind, mind is empty, emptiness has spontaneous existence, and that what is spontaneously existing is self-liberating" (Namgyal, 2019, p. 521), "which is the nature of bliss" (p. 520). As in these

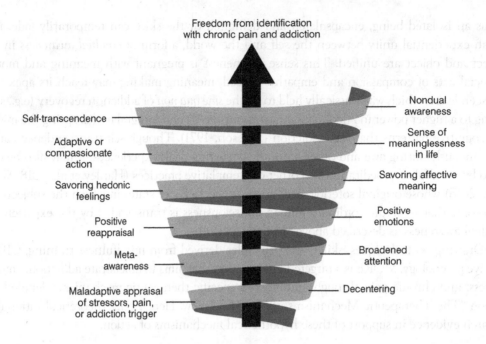

FIGURE 3.1. Upward spiral of mindfulness to meaning and self-transcendence. From "Mindfulness Broadens Awareness and Builds Eudaimonic Meaning" by E. L. Garland, N. A. Farb, P. R. Goldin, and B. L. Fredrickson. Copyright © 2015 Taylor & Francis. Adapted by permission.

Tibetan traditions, in MORE we assume some patients can, early on, achieve a "taste" of self-transcendence by simply directly pointing to the possibility that the observed (appearances) and the observer (mind) are one. Thus, such direct pointing instructions are even included in the basic mindful breathing practice introduced at the start of the program. Yet, we provide a fail-safe instruction ("You can focus on that part of the mind now, *or* you can continue to focus on the breathing") under the assumption that most patients will not be able to access a taste of self-transcendence in the first several MORE sessions. In our experience, some (but not all) patients do report meditation-induced experiences of oneness or a quieting of the sense of self by the end of the 8-week MORE program (Garland, Hanley, Hudak, et al., 2022; Garland, Hanley, Riquino, et al., 2019; Hudak et al., 2021). We discuss self-transcendence and nondual awareness in greater depth in Chapter 7.

MORE Treatment Program Basics

The MORE treatment program is an 8-week program consisting of mind–body skill practices revolving around mindfulness, reappraisal, savoring, and self-transcendence. Typically, participants meet once a week for 8 weeks, although MORE can also be delivered twice a week for 4 weeks—a format that may be more fitting for classic 30-day addiction treatment programs. MORE is typically delivered as a group therapy, although it can be delivered as an individual therapy as well. For the group version of MORE, each session is 2 hours long; for individual MORE, sessions are 55 minutes in length. Sessions follow a structured agenda. Because MORE was originally designed as a group therapy and the majority of research on MORE has been conducted on the group therapy version of the treatment, Sessions 1–8 present the structured agendas for the 2-hour group format of MORE. Note that it is possible to run a MORE group in 90-minute sessions, but that when doing so, the amount of processing time becomes significantly reduced. When delivering MORE as an individual therapy, each session can be structured with the following timeline: 15–20 minutes for the introductory mindfulness practice, followed by a 10- to 15-minute debrief (the PURER process outlined in Chapter 5), followed by 10 minutes of psychoeducation, with the concluding mind–body practice and debrief taking the remaining 15–20 minutes.

Participants are asked to practice homework each week, guided by handouts and mind–body skill recordings. Home practice consists of 15 minutes of mindfulness (mindful breathing and/or body scan) a day each week. After reappraisal is introduced in Session 3 and savoring in Session 4, participants are also asked to practice each of these skills one time a day. Participants may be able to complete a reappraisal practice session in a matter of minutes (though it could take longer, depending on how long the patient requires to go through the steps), whereas savoring should be practiced for 10–15 minutes at a time, ideally. It is optimal for you, as the MORE therapist, to generate your own meditation recordings for your patient. Because you have developed a positive, caring, therapeutic relationship with your own patients, they will respond more effectively to recordings of mind–body skill practice made by your own voice rather than the voice of a faceless stranger. I recommend that you record yourself delivering each of the primary mind–body skill techniques (i.e., mindful breathing, body scan, mindfulness of pain, savoring, mindfulness of craving). Most modern smartphones have a voice recorder app that can be used to record and email mind–body practice instructions to your patients; I have found this to provide a convenient solution with decent-enough sound quality.

Chapter 2 discussed how to identify whether the patient is a right fit for the MORE program. In terms of who is appropriate to serve as a MORE therapist, MORE should be delivered by a licensed or license-eligible health care provider. Social workers, psychologists, counselors, nurses, physicians (of a wide range of specialties), and even physical therapists have delivered MORE successfully. Besides being a compassionate clinician, you should have some basic knowledge of behavioral health treatment and assessment issues. Skills in building rapport, empathic responding, and active listening are basic prerequisites to delivering MORE. Similarly, a MORE therapist should have enough training in crisis management and de-escalation to deal with emotional decompensation during a session or posttraumatic flashbacks. Basic training in CBT is also extremely valuable when delivering MORE. You should also have a good grasp of the philosophy, science, and practice of mindfulness. As a starting place, I would recommend the classic text by Jon Kabat-Zinn (1990), *Full Catastrophe Living*, as well as *Mindfulness-Based Cognitive Therapy for Depression* (Segal et al., 2013) and the *Handbook of Mindfulness: Theory, Research, and Practice* (Brown et al., 2015). I encourage you to read review papers to get a sense of the neuroscience of mindfulness (e.g., Tang et al., 2015). For a basic, introductory philosophical–spiritual grounding, I recommend *What the Buddha Taught* (Rahula, 1959/2007), *Tao Te Ching* (Laozi & English, 2011), *The Sun My Heart* (Hanh, 1988), *Man's Search for Meaning* (Frankl, 1946/1959), and *The Book* (Watts, 1966/2011). For a more intense philosophical exploration, read *Mahāmudrā: the Moonlight-Quintessence of Mind and Meditation* (Namgyal, 2006) and *The Recognition Sutras* (Wallis, 2017).

Perhaps most importantly, to be a competent MORE therapist, having your own regular, disciplined mindfulness practice is essential. You do not need to be an expert meditator to deliver

MORE. You only need to have a little more experience than your patients to be helpful. However, you should commit to a daily practice of mindfulness while delivering MORE. Having such a practice will help you to understand, in a deeply experiential way, the states of consciousness and barriers your patients experience as they embark upon learning mindfulness. Armed with such an understanding, you will be a far more effective guide in helping your patients navigate the often challenging and confounding practice of mindfulness. In addition, having a daily mindfulness practice will help you embody the principles you are teaching in the MORE intervention. Without such a daily practice, your exhortations to your patients to regularly practice mindfulness will come across as phony and hypocritical.

> To be a competent MORE therapist, having your own mindfulness practice is essential.

MORE is a sequenced treatment (see Figure 3.2). It begins with a foundation of mindfulness training, which by virtue of its effects on enhancing attentional control and meta-awareness, is theorized to synergize therapeutic techniques that involve a greater degree of cognitive and emotional elaborative processing, like reappraisal and savoring. These treatment components aim to activate a series of therapeutic mechanisms, which are in turn intended to produce stepwise change in a range of clinical targets that are addressed sequentially as motivational ambivalence is resolved and patients become ready to alter their opioid use.

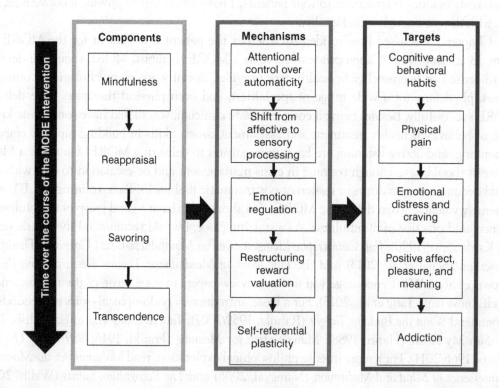

FIGURE 3.2. The MORE treatment sequence, its therapeutic mechanisms, and its treatment targets.

The Therapeutic Mechanisms of MORE

MORE Aims to Enhance Attentional Control over Automaticity

If, as Tiffany (1990) first proposed (see Chapter 2), addiction is an automatic habit controlled by drug use action schemas that operate outside of conscious awareness, then habitual use and misuse of opioids may be altered by using mindfulness to enhance awareness of activation of drug use action schema when triggered by substance-related cues or (emotional or physical) pain. Such conscious awareness may thereby allow for disruption of automatized drug use with a controlled coping response. For people with chronic substance use or those with substance use disorders, moderating or abstaining from drug use requires the deployment of conscious cognitive control mechanisms in stressful situations (Wiers et al., 2007). Classically, mindfulness meditation has been viewed as a means of de-automatization (Deikman, 1966)—the process whereby patterns of behavioral responses that had been rendered automatic and unconscious through repetition are reinvested with conscious attention. In light of evidence that mindfulness meditation increases access to unconscious processing (Fabbro et al., 2017; Strick et al., 2012) and disrupts habit responses (Greenberg et al., 2012; Hanley & Garland, 2019b; Wenk-Sormaz, 2005), MORE may increase awareness of automatic addictive tendencies and strengthen conscious control over them.

Given that drug use action schemas are triggered by cues associated with past episodes of substance use, the activation of these automatic addictive habits may be interrupted by shifting attention from substance-related triggers to neutral, positive, or health-promoting objects and events. As such, mindfulness involves practices that train sustained attention, attentional monitoring, and attentional reorienting capacity, in which the mindfulness practitioner (i.e., the patient) repeatedly places their attention onto an object (e.g., the sensation of breathing, the sensation of walking) while monitoring and accepting distracting thoughts and emotions, and then returning the attention back to the object of focus. Consequently, mindfulness has been construed as a means of attention regulation (Lutz et al., 2008). Indeed, meditation is associated with the strengthening of functional connectivity of the dorsal attentional network in the brain (Froeliger et al., 2012) and meta-analyses indicate that mindfulness augments attentional functions (Sumantry & Stewart, 2021). Specific to addiction, people with substance use disorders who are higher in trait mindfulness are better able to disengage their attention from addictive cues (Garland, Boettiger, et al., 2012) and to regulate their autonomic reactions to such cues (Baker & Garland, 2019; Garland, 2011). MORE offers training in disengaging attention from people, places, and things associated with past substance use (including internal body sensations stemming from stress and negative emotions) and refocusing on neutral or health-promoting stimuli, such as the sensation of one's own breath or a beautiful sunset. Over time, this practice may weaken linkages between substance-related cues and drug use action schema. Not surprisingly then, MORE has been shown to decrease attentional bias to opioid cues (Garland, Baker, et al., 2017; Garland, Nakamura, et al., 2024), coupled with decreased heart rate (Garland et al., 2014) and brain reactivity to opioid cues (Garland, Atchley, et al., 2019). In addition, through a similar approach of using mindfulness to engage and subsequently disengage attention from painful body sensations, MORE may reduce attentional hypervigilance toward pain, and indeed, MORE has been shown to decrease attentional bias toward pain-related information (Garland & Howard, 2013).

MORE Aims to Shift from Affective to Sensory Processing

As discussed in Chapter 2, people typically experience chronic pain as a monolithic, solid, and unremitting experience. Inferences and predictions derived from past pain episodes may result in biased interpretations of the body's current state that accumulate into maladaptive cognitive schemas that preserve and exacerbate pain. Thus, chronic pain often involves catastrophizing—that is, worrying and ruminating about body sensations as indicative of a worsening physical condition or a sign that pain will never go away. Furthermore, people with chronic pain experience sadness and anger from the losses they have experienced as a result of their pain. Such emotional anguish magnifies the pain experience.

To remedy this affective processing of pain, in MORE patients are instructed to practice mindfulness to remove this emotional overlay, and to "zoom in" (toward pain) and deconstruct unpleasant internal experiences (e.g., pain, craving, or negative emotions) into their constituent sensations (e.g., tightness, vibration, heat) while heightening awareness of the center, edges, and permeability (vs. solidity) of these sensations and noticing any proximal or distal pleasurable sensations. So rather than experiencing pain as some constant, terrible, awful anguish, patients are taught to reinterpret pain as harmless and impermanent sensations of tightness, or tingling, or heat, and to notice the spaces inside those sensations where there is no sensation at all, or potentially, even pleasant sensations embedded within or right next to the painful ones (Hanley & Garland, 2019a). Mindfully reinterpreting pain as pure sensation is consistent with the Buddhist *Abhidharma* tradition, which teaches mindful examination of phenomenological experience in a fine-grained manner to deconstruct and parse experiential gestalts into a transitory flux of cognitive, affective, and sensorial components (Nyanaponika, 1998). Moreover, the notion that pleasant sensation can exist contemporaneously with pain has parallels in Indo-Tibetan Tantric traditions, which provide instruction in the practice of mindful introspection of sensory experience, yielding the insight that all sensations, regardless of their valence, can be marked by the qualia of bliss (Dyczkowski, 1987; Tsongkhapa, 2012).

Using mindfulness to heighten interoceptive awareness and shift from affective to sensory processing of pain sensations may help to disrupt cognitive schemas of pain and reduce emotional bias during pain appraisals, thereby decreasing pain intensity and unpleasantness (Garland, 2020). And, we have found that this technique reduces

> Mindfully seeing pain as pure sensation decreases emotional anguish and makes pain hurt less.

postsurgical pain to a significantly greater extent than simple mindful breathing or CBT (Hanley et al., 2021). This practice of "zooming in" may reduce pain by helping the patient to sense the current physiological condition of their body, which may not be as unpleasant as their expectations and predictive models of pain (Wiech, 2016). Over time, this practice might reverse default mode, self-referential identification with pain discussed in Chapter 2.

MORE Aims to Regulate Negative Emotions and Craving

Given the role that negative emotions and craving play in priming pain and addictive behavior (Chapter 2), emotion regulation is a key therapeutic process in the treatment of people suffering from chronic pain, opioid misuse, and OUD. In that regard, many studies have demonstrated that mindfulness training can improve the ability to regulate negative emotions (Goyal et al., 2014; Leyland et al., 2019). Similarly, negative emotions can be powerfully addressed with cognitive restructuring, a CBT technique that challenges maladaptive appraisals of distressing life events and replaces them with alternative, more helpful ways of thinking (Beck et al., 1979). As discussed in "The Mindfulness-to-Meaning Theory" above, MORE provides training in a mindful reappraisal technique in which mindfulness is used to synergize cognitive restructuring. During the practice of mindful reappraisal, the person disengages from their initial negative appraisal into an open-minded state of meta-awareness in which thoughts and feelings are viewed as ephemeral mental events rather than accurate reflections of reality. In so doing, attention broadens to encompass a larger set of information from which one may generate new appraisals of the challenging life circumstance. By accessing this enlarged set of data pertaining to the situation, individuals can then more easily reappraise their circumstances as meaningful or growth promoting.

With regard to regulating craving, informed by Tiffany's (1990) cognitive processing model of addiction, MORE first aims to increase awareness of craving, and then to provide a means of dampening craving. According to the cognitive processing model, addictive behavior operates outside of awareness through the operation of automatic drug use action schemas when triggered by cues associated with past drug use episodes (e.g., the sight of a pill bottle or the feeling of physical or emotional pain). Consequently, many people struggling with misuse of prescription opioids may be wholly unaware of their addictive tendencies, and often deny experiencing opioid craving. This phenomenon is explicated by the cognitive processing model, which states that automatized drug use behaviors can occur in the absence of craving when access to drugs is unimpeded (such as at the beginning of a new 30-day prescription when one's pill bottle is full). Tiffany proposed that conscious craving occurs when an activated drug use action schema is blocked from reaching the goal of drug consumption. As such, persons in acute withdrawal, persons unable to obtain opioids (e.g., due to lack of money or tightening opioid prescription rules), or persons attempting to abstain from or moderate their use may experience an upwelling of craving. Without awareness of craving, the patient is likely to slip into automatized drug use, even in the absence of a conscious intention to use, and may unwittingly remain in high-risk situations and thus be especially vulnerable to relapse (Rohsenow et al., 1994).

Insofar as mindfulness enhances access to unconscious material, and promotes interoceptive awareness, MORE teaches the practice of mindfulness before using opioids as a means of helping the patient to realize when their opioid use is being driven by craving rather than by the need for relief of physical pain. Next, through a technique that parallels the mindfulness-of-pain technique described in the "Shift from Affective to Sensory Processing" section above, MORE teaches patients to "zoom in" and deconstruct craving into its cognitive, affective, and sensory components. This "zooming-in" practice facilitates craving exposure and extinction, while helping the patient to titrate their arousal and prevent flooding via mindful breathing and decentering. Following this "zooming-in" practice, MORE teaches reappraisal as a means of coping with craving, by guiding the patient to contemplate the consequences of indulging in drug use versus abstaining from use—a technique that has been shown to increase prefrontal regulation of drug cue–reactivity in the striatum (Kober et al., 2010). These dual, complementary practices of mindfulness and reappraisal provide a potent means of regulating craving, and indeed, MORE's craving-reducing effects have been demonstrated in multiple controlled trials (Parisi et al., 2022).

MORE Aims to Restructure Reward Processing

The downward spiral linking chronic pain to opioid misuse and OUD involves hedonic dysregulation, in which the individual becomes increasingly sensitive to cues representing drug-related rewards while becoming insensitive to the pleasure and meaning derived from naturally rewarding objects and events (see Chapter 2). Given this pathogenic process, MORE uses mindfulness to strengthen cognitive control and thereby facilitate reappraisal of opioid misuse as a source of adverse consequences and to savor natural, healthful stimuli as a source of pleasure, positive emotions, and meaning in life. When integrated with mindfulness training, these techniques represent complex sequences of emotion regulatory strategies aimed at restructuring reward processing from valuation of drug reward toward increased valuation of nondrug rewards. This therapeutic focus accords with my *restructuring reward hypothesis*, which states that shifting valuation from drug-related rewards back to natural rewards will reduce craving and addictive behavior (Garland, 2016, 2021). This restructuring reward process is the key by which MORE treats addiction.

Hypothetically, this restructuring of reward processing may arise from restoration of the feedback loop between prefrontal brain structures essential to cognitive control, and corticostriatal circuits crucial to reward learning and motivation (Garland, Froeliger, et al., 2013). In MORE, an integration of mindfulness, reappraisal, and savoring is used to facilitate restructuring of the perceived value of drug- and non-drug-related rewards and reconfigure their meaning in relation to the self. With respect to opioids, this process entails changing one's relationship to the drug from one in which it is appraised as a source of immediate gratification to one in which the drug represents delayed negative consequences. With respect to natural rewards, this process entails changing one's relationship to the simple pleasures and positive experiences in daily life from being comparatively less salient (i.e., anhedonia, the consequence of addiction-related reward processing impairments) to being a powerful source of reward and a deep source of personal meaning. The therapeutic process of restructuring reward learning may be an essential mechanism of recovery from opioid misuse and addiction. The person in recovery must relearn what is and what is not important in life, reclaiming the sense of meaning that was hijacked by the addictive process and reinvesting it back into the people, activities, and values they once cared about.

> MORE treats addiction by restructuring reward processing from valuing drug-related rewards back to valuing natural, healthy rewards.

To do so, MORE teaches a mindful savoring technique in which mindfulness is used to attend to and savor the pleasant sensory features (i.e., visual, auditory, olfactory, gustatory, tactile) of naturally rewarding objects and events (e.g., a beautiful landscape, social affiliation), as well as the positive emotions and sensations that flow from them (Garland, 2016). When the patient becomes aware of these feelings, they are guided to turn their attention inward, and savor the positive inner feeling. By cultivating meta-awareness of the resultant positive emotional state, higher-order affective meanings may arise (Garland & Fredrickson, 2019)—for instance, the sense that one's self has worth and life itself has value—resulting in gratitude and compassion. In this way, mindful savoring enhances the hedonic and eudaimonic dimensions of well-being (Garland, Farb, et al., 2015b). When positive emotions and affective associations begin to fade, attention shifts outward again to appreciating the pleasant object or event. Hypothetically (as discussed in the "Savoring" section above), this toggling of exteroceptive and interoceptive attention on pleasant perceptions, sensations, cognitions, emotions, and memories may overcome the "hedonic treadmill effect" (Brickman & Campbell, 1971) to prolong and intensify the positive experience.

In that regard, MORE has been shown to amplify physiological responsiveness to natural rewards, as evidenced by increased autonomic nervous system (Garland et al., 2014) and brain activation (Froeliger et al., 2017; Garland et al., 2023; Garland, Atchley, et al., 2019; Garland, Froeliger, et al., 2015b) in response to natural reward images (e.g., smiling babies, beautiful sunsets, lovers holding hands). In turn, this increased responsiveness to natural rewards accounted for MORE's effects on reducing craving and opioid misuse (Garland et al., 2014; Garland, Atchley, et al., 2019; Garland, Howard, et al., 2017), demonstrating that MORE treats addiction by restructuring reward valuation, reversing the allostatic process, and helping the patient to relearn what is and what is not meaningful in life.

Through the integration of mindfulness meditation and savoring, the patient may learn to self-generate a sense of bliss (Garland, 2021; Garland & Fredrickson, 2019). Although the exact neurobiological mechanisms of this process remain unknown, meditative self-generation of hedonic pleasure and ecstatic states are likely underpinned by activation in corticostriatal circuits implicated in reward and undergirded by increased endogenous dopamine and opioid release (Hagerty et al., 2013; Sharp, 2014), not unlike the neurochemical release occasioned by drug use itself (Spagnolo et al., 2019). From this perspective, inducing pleasant sensations through meditative practices can provide a safe, nonaddictive, and nondrug means of reward—a "natural high" and endogenous form of self-stimulation (Olds & Milner, 1954) that may replace the craving for drug-induced reward.

MORE Aims to Induce Self-Referential Plasticity

The therapeutic process of MORE may reach its apex in self-transcendence—classically held to be the *sine qua non* of addiction recovery (e.g., surrendering to a higher power in AA). This sense of connecting to something greater than the self may involve a radical shift in self-awareness and the sense of one's own identity. As discussed in Chapter 2, both chronic pain and addiction often lead to maladaptive forms of identification, wherein events in life are processed with reference to their relevance to autobiographical narratives of pain and drug use. Rather than being immersed in egocentricity and feelings of isolation that both fuel and result from addiction, through self-transcendent states produced during meditation one may come to experience the self as being open, expansive, and interdependent (see Chapter 7), connected to others and the world at large. In that regard, we have found that the self-transcendent states produced by the core MORE mindfulness meditation practice are linked with increased theta EEG activity in frontal midline brain regions that promotes significant reductions in opioid use and misuse (Garland, Hanley, Hudak, et al., 2022; Hudak et al., 2021). Instead of being plagued by painful feelings of lack, an insatiable craving and grasping, and a gaping hole that one constantly scrambles to fill with addictive behavior, through self-transcendence one realizes their fundamental identity with the whole of life, which leads to a sense of fullness and completion. By recognizing this deep interconnectedness or fundamental unity between the self and the world, the self is transformed, the meaning of one's life begins to shift, and out of this shift may arise a deep and abiding selfless motivation to help others in need and act in the service of compassion. Ultimately, meditative self-transcendence may engender a durable form of stimulus-independent happiness, undergirded by increased functional connectivity among intrinsic and extrinsic brain networks implicated in processing the self and the external world (Garland, 2021).

In summary, MORE's multicomponent treatment approach is designed to target an array of therapeutic mechanisms intended to produce positive clinical outcomes relevant to people recovering from chronic pain, opioid misuse, and addiction. MORE was developed by taking discoveries from the basic behavioral science and neuroscience of addiction and chronic pain, and translating those discoveries into specific, actionable techniques, tools, and psychological technologies that can be used to strengthen recovery, alleviate suffering, and amplify human flourishing. In the next chapter, we discuss how mindfulness, as the foundation of MORE, should be delivered to maximize the healing potential of this ancient and powerful technique in the context of the MORE therapy.

Chapter 4

Anatomy of a Mindfulness Meditation

MORE starts with the basic philosophy that the therapeutic session is not merely an opportunity for psychoeducation. Rather, the session itself should provide the patient with a healing experience. When you teach mindfulness, reappraisal, and savoring skills to the patient, you are not only trying to impart a skill but even more so trying to help heal your patient. As articulated in Chapter 1, MORE is founded on a recovery-oriented framework that presupposes that the patient has the inner resources to heal and reclaim a meaningful life from chronic pain, emotional distress, and addictive behavior. While the mind–body has the intrinsic capacity to heal itself, the clinician can stimulate the healing process through the skillful use of therapeutic tools. Physicians heal through tools, including medication and surgical instruments. As a MORE therapist, you have no such material tools. Instead, you facilitate the healing of your patient through your communications, both verbal and nonverbal. Your therapeutic tools are your voice, your gestures, and your facial expressions. You use these tools to affect a change in your patient's thoughts, emotions, behaviors, and body sensations.

Therefore, you should think of teaching mindfulness (and reappraisal and savoring) not as teaching a skill but rather as a process of imparting therapeutic suggestions to the client (Yapko, 2011, 2020). When one practices mindfulness meditation (or reappraisal or savoring) on one's own, without active guidance by a therapist, this form of individual practice involves the internal self-regulation of attention, affect, cognition, and physiology, without any use of suggestions. In contrast, when a therapist provides mindfulness instruction to a patient, they are delivering suggestions to stimulate changes in the patient's psychological experience and bodily state (not unlike hypnosis). From this perspective, every instruction you provide, every sentence you speak, is actually a suggestion for activating various cognitive-affective processes, altering your patient's state of awareness, and modifying the contents of their consciousness—whether you realize it or not![1]

Carefully consider the possible impact of your suggestions with regard to their potential to elicit a healing response in your patient. In this sense, MORE is a strategic therapy approach. Ask yourself continuously, "What am I trying to accomplish with this communication?" This high

---

[1] In this sense, the development of MORE is indebted to the work of Milton Erickson, a virtuoso psychotherapist who pioneered the use of indirect suggestion in hypnotherapy (Erickson et al., 1976).

degree of intentionality will increase the parsimony, precision, and efficacy of your approach, leading to better clinical outcomes.

It is not only what you say but how you say it that matters. Receptivity to suggestions can be increased under conditions of heightened rapport. Rapport is produced not only by genuine empathy and unconditional positive regard for the patient. Rapport can also be generated unconsciously through synchrony. *Synchrony* is the process whereby two natural systems, which have different action patterns when they function independently, become entrained to each other by oscillating at a shared vibratory frequency (or resonance). Examples from nature include when two swinging pendulums begin to swing together to the same rhythm, a flying bird joins a flock and flies in perfect coordination with it, crickets chirp in unison in a chorus, fireflies flash their light displays at the same time, and women who live together begin to share a common menstrual cycle. Synchrony also occurs in social interactions (Hoehl et al., 2021), and reverberates from physical to psychological levels, resulting in an increased sense of rapport between individuals. Take for example the famous experiment by John Bargh and Tanya Chartrand (Chartrand & Bargh, 1999). Research subjects were sent to a room to have a conversation with a research assistant about a photograph. With half of the subjects, the research assistant maintained a neutral body position. For the other subjects, the research assistant mimicked the posture, mannerisms, and movements of the subject. So, every time a subject crossed their legs, the research assistant crossed their legs. Every time a subject touched their hair, the research assistant touched their hair. At the end of the experiment, subjects were asked to rate how much they liked their research assistant. Subjects whose movements had been mirrored rated their research assistants as more likable and the interaction as being smoother than subjects whose research assistants did not mirror body language. However, no subject was aware that the mirroring had occurred—it had been performed outside of their awareness. Unconscious mirroring increases the sense of trust and openness to suggestion. The mirroring of communications (both verbal and nonverbal) is a tactic often used in persuasion; skilled salespeople use this tactic to get you to buy more expensive things than you ever intended to buy (think back to the last time you bought a car).

> It is not just what you say but how you say it that matters.

In MORE, we leverage this principle in multiple ways. For instance, we can create rapport by pacing our rate of speech to the patient's breathing rate during mindfulness instruction. Each time the patient breathes in, we provide a verbal suggestion—for example, "You can notice the sensation of the breath moving into the nostrils." And when the patient breathes out, we offer the next suggestion. In so doing, we induce a form of synchrony that may remain unconscious for the patient, but nevertheless creates the impression that the clinician is "with the patient" and "in sync." Such synchrony is fairly easy to establish when working with an individual patient by attending to the rise and fall of the patient's chest, diaphragm, or abdomen. However, when working with a group of individuals all breathing at different rates, this tactic can be managed by dividing your mindfulness instruction time up by pacing your suggestions to a few breaths of each patient in the group. In this way, each patient may feel that you are "with them"—despite your delivery of mindfulness to the entire group.

Similarly, we leverage synchrony when strategically modulating vocal tone and pacing during mindfulness instruction to affect the patient's emotional state. Think of the way a masterful orator, actor, or singer can captivate an entire audience, bringing them to tears or cries of joy through the power of their voice and the dramatic use of silence. When providing mindfulness instruction, typically we aim to use a tone similar to that one would use to soothe a baby. When babies cry out of anxiety or frustration, parents use a soothing, hushed voice to suggest relaxation and calm, coupled with physical affection—a gentle touch that produces pleasure and releases muscle tension. When repeated over time, the soothing tone becomes a conditioned stimulus that elicits a conditioned relaxation response, such that a mere "shhhh" can lull a crying baby into quiescence. As adults, we unconsciously retain this early patterning. Using a soothing voice when teaching mindfulness may elicit this conditioned response, increasing the relaxing and calming effects of the meditation. That said, there may be moments when you would rather emphasize feelings of clarity, wakefulness, or alertness over relaxation and calm. If so, using a crisp, clear vocal inflection may help to impart this feeling state. Strategically modulating vocal tone between soothing and crisp phrasings over the course of a meditation session can create unconscious emphases on particular suggestions, potentially accentuating their impact.

With regard to pacing, we attend not only to the frequency with which we speak words, phrases, and sentences, and the spaces in between those utterances but also to the length of each syllable. Speaking slowly, with space between words, is another means of suggesting calm and relaxation. Perhaps even more importantly, it is critically important to give the patient adequate time to follow the suggestions you are offering. After each suggestion you provide, the patient must engage a range of cognitive processes in order to experience what you are suggesting. Many of the suggestions you provide are complex and unusual (e.g., "Are there spaces inside the sensation where the sensation is not?"). How much time does it take to follow each suggestion? You can use your own experience as a barometer to make this determination. With each suggestion you provide, you should stop, turn your attention inward, and follow your own suggestion. In other words, you should be practicing mindfulness yourself as you provide your patients with mindfulness instruction. This will allow you to roughly estimate the amount of time it will take for your patient to follow the suggestion. That said, if you are an experienced meditator, you might need to add several seconds of silence after you follow your own suggestion, under the assumption that due to your meditation experience you can engage the requisite cognitive processes more rapidly than can your patient. Another purpose of following your own suggestions is for reasons of authenticity and synchrony. It is possible (though as yet unsubstantiated by empirical data) that the extent to which you can immerse yourself in presence and meta-awareness while providing meditation instruction may affect your patient's ability to immerse themselves in presence and meta-awareness during mindfulness practice. If you meditate with deep concentration or open awareness, it may help your patient achieve deep concentration or open awareness during meditation. Recent dyadic neuroimaging research indicates that the oscillatory activity of human brains exhibits synchrony when people are communicating with one another (Kelsen et al., 2020). Plausibly, such synchrony occurs during mindfulness practice as well, as transmitted through verbal and nonverbal communications during the deep rapport developed by a therapist closely aligning with the patient.

The silent spaces between suggestions should also be increased incrementally across the weekly MORE sessions. You may note that the text for the guided mindfulness of pain practice each week is the same, yet the length of time devoted to each practice session is increased each week. How is this possible? We elongate each session not by adding words *but by adding silence*. We upwardly titrate the length of the spaces between suggestions to the growing ability of the patient to handle silence. Do not underestimate how difficult silence may be for patients, especially those who have been victims of past trauma, or those facing serious present life adversity. Silence may be the stimulus for flashbacks, rumination, or worrying about the future. It is important to give the patient the time and space to process and self-regulate these issues internally using the mind–body skills you are teaching, but only when they have developed a sufficient foundation of coping techniques and self-regulation strength to navigate the silence without becoming overwhelmed. To keep your patients from drowning in silence, you can use your voice to "throw them a lifeline." In the midst of the long silent spaces of mindfulness practice in Sessions 6–8, you can interject simple statements like "Just noticing where the mind is in this moment. Is it focused on the breath, or wandering? And wherever the mind is, that's okay. Just noticing where the mind is, acknowledging and accepting that experience, then letting it go, and bringing your attention back to the breath." After making these suggestions, you can return to an elongated period of silence.

In contrast, using a staccato, fast voice tone suggests tension, stress, and rapid mind wandering, while simultaneously preventing the patient from actually following each suggestion in time. Consequently, the patient has the experience of rushing to follow suggestions that may be perceived as confusing and quickly forgotten, leaving the patient with the impression that

> From one session to the next, increase the silent spaces between suggestions.

"mindfulness just doesn't work for me." Therefore, I strongly recommend practicing delivering the guided meditation practices and recording your voice, so you can critically evaluate the quality of your tone and pacing. In addition, because patients develop a rapport and therapeutic relationship with you, providing them with recordings of your voice leading mind–body skill practice, to use at home between sessions, may be more effective than using generic recordings made by others.

Finally, it is crucial to remain attuned to the therapy context while guiding mindfulness practice—that is, to preserve synchrony and rapport, you should be responsive to your patients' experience. If the patient begins to cry during mindfulness practice, you might say,

"Soon you may begin to notice that the mind begins to wander to thoughts, or feelings, maybe even strong feelings. And if the mind wanders to strong feelings, that's okay, that's what minds do, they wander. You can just notice where the mind has wandered, and acknowledge and accept that feeling, telling yourself in the space of your own mind, it's okay to have this strong feeling right now, and then you can let it go, and gently but firmly return the focus of the attention back to the breath."

Similarly, if there is a loud banging in the hallway outside the therapy room or noises that occur in the group like coughing, cell phones ringing, or the shuffling of chairs, you could say,

"Soon you may notice that the mind begins to wander to thoughts, or sounds, maybe even loud sounds. And if the mind wanders to sounds, that's okay, that's what minds do, they wander. You can just notice where the mind has wandered, and acknowledge and accept that sound, telling yourself in the space of your own mind, it's okay to hear this sound right now, and then you can let it go, and gently but firmly return the focus of the attention back to the breath."

The same tactic can be used to address a patient who has begun to snore (" . . . the mind begins to wander to feelings of sleepiness . . . "), or laugh (" . . . the mind begins to wander to feeling like you want to laugh, or thoughts like 'this is silly or weird' . . . "), or experience any other potential barrier to practice. The principle here is to "roll with the resistance" (Miller, 1983) and to fold in whatever experience arises in the moment as a practice opportunity. In so doing, your guidance becomes alive and dynamically integrated with all that the therapy moment has to offer, rather than being some fossilized script whose delivery is out of sync with the patient's lived experience.

> Keep your guidance alive and integrated with whatever arises in the moment.

Many mindfulness teachers are unaware of the aforementioned strategies for enhancing rapport and synchrony. That said, I think the great mindfulness teachers intuitively engage in these strategies. You don't have to be a naturally adept mindfulness teacher. Instead, through practice and conscious strategic effort, you can be a great mindfulness teacher for your patients by leveraging the principles described above (i.e., voice tone, pacing, silence, attunement, suggestion).

Again, if you practice mindfulness at the same time that you are providing mindfulness instruction, these tactics will be less contrived, and more authentic, emerging out of your openness and sensitive contact to the present moment during the therapy experience. Of course, it is natural for your attention to drift during therapy, as your own mind wanders due to unconscious associations that are triggered during the session. Furthermore, when the mindfulness meditations become longer over the course of the eight sessions of MORE, your own mind is likely to wander during the silent periods of the mindfulness instruction. This can result in you becoming lost and losing your place in delivering the guided meditation practice. These are additional reasons why it is imperative for you to have a solid and regular mindfulness practice when you are delivering MORE. With a regular mindfulness practice, your attention is more likely to remain stable and focused during the session, and you will be able to catch yourself more quickly when your mind begins to wander. But, if you do lose contact with the present moment during the session, you should embody the principles you are trying to teach, and adopt a nonjudgmental attitude toward yourself while returning your attention back to your own breath for one or two breathing cycles, before reorienting your attention back to delivering the guided meditation practice or therapeutic content for the session.

Mindfulness Instruction as Suggestion

Following the principles just set forth, consider mindfulness instruction as a process of using suggestion to help your patient activate therapeutic cognitive and emotional mechanisms to evoke a range of desired experiential responses. These different experiential responses can be emphasized or de-emphasized, according to specific client needs and individual differences. By becoming aware of the underlying structure of a mindfulness meditation, a therapist implementing MORE can be more intentional and strategic in their approach with patients. Furthermore, the therapist may feel a greater freedom to modify the guided meditation or improvise in the moment by using different words, phrases, and metaphors to accomplish the same therapeutic ends. This is important, because it allows you to dynamically adjust your suggestions to the concepts, ideas, and metaphors most personally meaningful to the patient. In the text that follows, instructions for the mindfulness-of-pain technique are presented, along with the rationale for each separate instruction.

The 10 steps in the list that follows here outline the underlying anatomy of suggestions embedded in the MORE mindfulness meditation.

1. *Providing rationale and building positive expectancy*—explaining why mindfulness is a logical solution to the patient's problems, providing information about the benefits of mindfulness (including research findings), and promoting the positive expectation that the patient will be successful in learning mindfulness and that doing so will alleviate their symptoms. This occurs outside of mindfulness meditation practice, throughout the didactic portion of MORE sessions (as well as in the education/expectancy step of PURER, described in Chapter 5).

2. *Focusing attention on the object of mindfulness*—directing the patient to orient their attention to an object of focus while suspending thoughts and mental "to-do" lists during the mindfulness practice session. Objects of mindfulness can include the sensation of the breath moving into one's nostrils or deeper in the lungs, other body sensations, external sensory targets, or, for more advanced practitioners, the field of awareness itself.

3. *Monitoring experience with meta-awareness*—instructing the patient to remain focused on the object of mindfulness while monitoring the field of awareness to notice the arising of mental contents other than the intended object (i.e., mind wandering). When mental contents other than the object of mindfulness are noted, examining them from the perspective of an observer or witness can generate insight into the nature of all experience as transitory and potentially marked by the qualia of emptiness and bliss (Dyczkowski, 1987; Tsongkhapa, 2012).

4. *Accepting whatever arises*—guiding the patient to allow mental contents to arise, change, and fade away without self-blame, condemnation, clinging, or resistance. Acceptance also involves adopting a form of self-compassion or loving-kindness toward one's own reactivity to whatever experience arises during mindfulness practice.

5. *Returning attention back to the object of mindfulness*—directing the patient to disengage or "let go" of their attention from unintended thoughts, emotions, sensations, and perceptions, and reorient their focus back to the intended object of mindfulness.

Steps 2–5 represent what we call in MORE the *loop of mindfulness* (see Handout S1.2). Although many patients (and therapists) wrongly believe that mindfulness is only Step 2 (focusing attention on the object of mindfulness), in actuality, the totality of these steps represents the process of mindfulness. With each iteration of the loop of mindfulness, one is strengthening the capacity for meta-awareness. When viewed from this perspective, the inevitable mind wandering that occurs during mindfulness practice represents a practice opportunity, as is stated in the meditation itself, "Each time the mind wanders, and you notice where it wanders off to and you acknowledge and accept that experience and you let it go, you are learning to step back into the open space of mindfulness." Understanding and communicating this concept effectively during the processing of mindfulness (discussed in Chapter 5) will lead to your patients feeling more successful and empowered in their ability to practice mindfulness.

> With each iteration of the loop of mindfulness, one is strengthening the capacity for meta-awareness.

6. *Utilization of mindfulness for symptom relief*—suggesting how the patient can use the processes activated during the loop of mindfulness to alleviate particular symptoms. For instance, utilization occurs when one guides the patient to use attentional control and acceptance to zoom in and out from pain and craving.

7. *Decentering*—providing instruction in the use of meta-awareness to "step back" and gain psychological distance from mental contents, and in so doing, viewing them not as immutable "facts" but instead as ever-changing mental experiences occurring within the larger field or space of awareness. Decentering helps a patient to disengage from problems/symptoms to allow for the final stages of the mindfulness practice.

8. *Self-transcendence*—offering the possibility that meta-awareness can deepen to the point that the distinction between observer and observed may momentarily fade or disappear completely while wakeful consciousness is maintained. The self-transcendent state may be marked by qualia of openness, vastness, clarity, luminosity, and freedom (Metzinger, 2024; Namgyal, 2006, 2019).

9. *Savoring*—directing the patient to notice, appreciate, and enjoy the positive emotions, pleasant body sensations, and meaningful insights that arise during mindfulness meditation without attachment or clinging. The patient can also be guided to appreciate the most "useful" or therapeutic parts of the meditative experience (which can be appropriate even in cases when meditation does not produce positive feelings).

10. *Ending the meditation*—instructing the patient to bring their practice to a close while building the positive expectancy that repeated practice will deepen the state of mindfulness in the future.

To clarify, the suggestions above, although described linearly, are actually often presented in a recursive fashion—that is, the basic loop of mindfulness (Steps 2–5) can be repeated to extend the length of the mindfulness session. Also, during silent periods of practice or any other appropriate moment in the session (e.g., after a loud noise, after the patient exhibits a strong emotional response), you may invite the patient to refocus their attention to the object of mindfulness (e.g., the sensation of breathing) or to accept the arising of unintended (and undesired) thoughts, emotions, and body sensations. Moreover, the loop of mindfulness is embedded within Step 6, insofar as coping with pain and craving via "zooming in" and "zooming out" involves focused attention, meta-awareness, acceptance, attentional reorienting, and decentering. Table 4.1 illustrates how each of these types of suggestions are embedded into the MORE mindfulness-of-pain practice.

To conclude, teaching and learning mindfulness in MORE involves a deep process of attunement, in which the therapist develops a sensitive awareness to verbal and nonverbal communications with the patient, a form of synchrony that leads to the resonance between two minds needed to open receptivity to therapeutic suggestion. In turn, this process activates the mechanisms of mindfulness by which the patient may leverage their own inherent potential for healing and psychological growth. But the healing process does not end with the practice of mindfulness. Instead, lasting growth comes from investigating and honoring the experiences that arise during mindfulness (and the other mind–body practices in MORE). This is where the magic of MORE happens. Chapter 5 describes this approach in detail.

TABLE 4.1. The Underlying Anatomy of Suggestions Embedded in the MORE Mindfulness Meditation Script

Providing rationale and building positive expectancy	*Mindfulness can help you to turn down the volume of your pain. Science shows that mindfulness can actually decrease the intensity of pain.*
Focusing attention on the object of mindfulness	*And when you are ready, you can begin to notice the sensation of the breath moving into the nostrils . . . and there's no need to breathe in any sort of special way. . . . Just noticing the natural sensation of the breath. . . . Noticing the temperature of that air . . . its warmth or coolness. . . .*
Monitoring experience with meta-awareness	*And soon you may notice that the mind begins to wander. . . . It may have already wandered . . . to thoughts, emotions, images, memories, or sensations.*
Accepting whatever arises	*Just noticing where the mind has wandered off to . . . acknowledging . . . and accepting that thought or feeling. . . . You might even say to yourself, "It's okay to have this experience right now, whatever it is. . . ."*
Returning attention back to the object of mindfulness	*And then, you can let it go. . . . and then gently, but firmly, bring the attention back to the sensation of the breath moving into the nostrils . . . back to the sensation of the breath moving deeper in the lungs. . . .*
Utilization of mindfulness for symptom relief	*And now imagine that you can breathe right into those sensations. . . . Imagining that you can send your breath right into those sensations, to soften them, like water seeping down into soil. . . .*
Decentering	*You are learning to step back . . . to step back . . . to step back from your thoughts and feelings and into the clear, open space of mindfulness. . . .*
Self-transcendence	*But there is a deeper part of the mind . . . that is more like . . . the space in which the clouds pass . . . the observing awareness . . . that is open . . . vast . . . perfect . . . and free . . . just watching, just observing. . . .*
Savoring	*And now, you can take a few long moments to focus on whatever positive experiences have come up for you during this practice . . . Appreciating and savoring those experiences now. . . .*

Chapter 5

Processing Mindfulness in a PURER Way

The true power of the MORE therapeutic approach stems from how we debrief and process the patient's practice of mindfulness, reappraisal, and savoring skills. The MORE processing approach is exquisitely important for helping the patient to consolidate what they have learned from the mind–body skill practice, and then to help them generalize that learning into coping with their symptoms of chronic pain, emotional distress, and opioid misuse in everyday life. The overarching principle here, informed by solution-focused therapy (de Shazer, 1988), is to search for exceptions to the patients' suffering by *focusing on positive* (i.e., *therapeutic*) *experience*. This orientation toward positive experience differs from the nondirective approach to inquiry used in other mindfulness teaching traditions. This difference is by design. Given that many patients with chronic pain and addiction suffer from negative cognitive biases and schemas of worthlessness (see Chapter 2), they are attuned to their failures and shortcomings, and overlook (or actively discount) their successes. An explicit and directive focus on positive experience is an important remedy to these patients' pessimistic default mode. Moreover, a focus on positive experience during processing can counter the reward deficits integral to opioid misuse and OUD (see Chapter 2) via an implicit form of savoring. During the savoring implicit to the MORE processing approach, the patient is guided through the therapist's questions to engage in positive rumination (Feldman et al., 2008) on moments during the mind–body skill practice when they felt good, experienced symptom relief, or realized some degree of psychological growth. During processing, you should ask yourself continuously, "How can I use this example or discussion point to teach, emphasize, or reinforce the concepts and skills I am trying to impart?" I use the acronym PURER to describe this processing approach: phenomenology, utilization, reframing, education/expectancy, and reinforcement. PURER also serves as a nice mnemonic to help you to remember what to do when processing:

Phenomenological—break patient experience down into clear steps that they and other group members can follow; focus on positive experiences

Utilization—help the patient to identify how they can use this experience and learning for coping in everyday life

Reframing—transform the patient's report into an example of what you are trying to teach

Education and expectancy—give more information about the phenomena experienced during the mind–body practice; build expectancy that positive effects will increase

Reinforcement—encourage and support practice and success experiences

The MORE treatment program uses PURER in processing the patient's experience of mind–body skill practice in each session and to process the patient's experience of mind–body skill practice for homework.

Although the acronym PURER implies a temporal sequence, the PURER techniques can and should be used in any sequence that makes sense given the patient's ongoing report of their experience during the mind–body practice. Typically, we begin with P (phenomenology). But U (utilization) may not immediately follow. To the contrary, often P is followed by R (reinforcement) or E (education). Moreover, the PURER techniques are often implemented in recursive loops, such that the therapist may get phenomenological, or provide education or reinforcement multiple times within a given processing effort with a given patient.

When processing mind–body skill practice, we always begin with the same question prompt: "What did you like best about this experience?" (or, with respect to homework practice, a variant like "What went well for you this week when you practiced mindfulness?"). This question carries an important indirect suggestion and implication: that there was some success experience or something of therapeutic value that occurred during the practice experience. Axiomatically, we assume mind–body skill practice is therapeutic and will result in some sort of beneficial experience for the patient. By asking the question in this way, this process of inquiry initiates a *transderivational* search (Grinder et al., 1977): an internal scanning of memories and associations that requires the patient to process their inner experience intensely to derive personally relevant meaning from the experience. The question "What did you like best?" directs the patient to identify and focus on positive experience. This type of loaded question is in contrast to an open-ended type of inquiry ("So, tell me about your experience"), which might elicit immediate negative reports ("That was awful! I hate mindfulness. It doesn't work for me!") from vocal group members with negative cognitive biases that could damage rapport and enthusiasm in the group, and put the therapist on the defensive. If a patient starts with a complaint or negative report in response to the question "What did you like best?," gently redirect back to success experience, with a statement such as "It sounds like that was a challenging experience. What you said is very important, and I really want to address challenges, but we are going to talk about that next. First, let's start with what people liked best about the experience." When the patient describes what they liked best, the next step is to engage in the PURER process to unpack that therapeutic experience in order to consolidate and reinforce the learning from that experience.

> Start with what patients liked best about the practice.

Once patients have described "what they liked best," the next question prompt to be asked is "Did you experience anything challenging about that experience?" Notice, whereas the first prompt, "What did you like best?" carries an implication that there was something the patient liked best about the experience, the second prompt carries no such implication and allows for the possibility that the patient will deny any challenging experiences. It is quite possible that no challenges occurred and the patient enjoyed the experience fully. If patients do not report challenges, move on to the next part of the session. In contrast to the therapeutic experiences described above, we do not assume the mind–body practice was challenging but we do want to honor difficult experiences. As in Rumi's (1995) poem "The Guest House," instances of physical or emotional pain, worries, regrets, and traumatic memories are welcome guests. "This being human is a guest house. Every morning a new arrival. A joy, a depression, a meanness. . . . Welcome and entertain them all!" (p. 109). Any reports of challenges should be responded to with the PURER approach, to reframe those challenges as learning opportunities (see "Reframing" below), help the patient identify a successful experience despite of the challenge, and provide education as needed to help troubleshoot or normalize the experience.

Let's explore the components of the PURER acronym in detail now.

Phenomenology

The first step in the PURER process is to get phenomenological. Phenomenology is an approach that focuses on the details of one's own conscious experience. The term *phenomenology* stems from a philosophical movement founded by philosophers including Husserl, Heidegger, and Merleau-Ponty in the first half of the 20th century. Phenomenology consists of systematic reflection on "lived experience" as a means of revealing the structures of consciousness and the phenomena that appear during acts of consciousness. In this sense, mindfulness itself might be construed as a form of phenomenological inquiry (Varela et al., 1991). With this consideration in mind, getting phenomenological is the primary means of accessing a patient's experience during their mindfulness practice (and practice of the other mind–body skills in MORE). Given its primacy and central importance to the therapeutic process, phenomenology is the first letter in the PURER acronym.

Before we discuss the "how" to getting phenomenological, we must first discuss why phenomenology is so important, and what our goal is in getting phenomenological with a patient's experience. Each mindfulness meditation practice session is a complex experience that reveals subtle layers of thought, emotion, and sensation. Sometimes the patient may access mental contents that are difficult to comprehend. Often, the states of consciousness evoked during mindfulness meditation are fleeting and unfamiliar to novice meditators. Their ephemerality and unfamiliarity make such altered states difficult to grasp and understand. Yet, despite their elusive quality, these states of consciousness can have significant therapeutic potential—for example, our research has demonstrated that experiencing self-transcendent states of consciousness during mindfulness meditation is linked with reduced pain and opioid misuse (Garland, Hanley, Hudak, et al., 2022; Garland, Hanley, Riquino, et al., 2019). Encouraging the patient to try to put their experience into words can enable them to discriminate the subtle aspects of experience that might have otherwise gone unnoticed.

Phenomenology is important for helping the patient to recognize, appreciate, and savor the therapeutic experiences arising during mind–body skill practice. As outlined in Chapter 3, savoring is an essential therapeutic mechanism of MORE in that it activates the reward system and generates motivational energy for positive change. By getting the patient to reflect on and talk about, in great detail, their positive experiences during mindfulness practice, this active review allows the patient to relish and relive those experiences a second time, providing another opportunity to engage in savoring, as described above. Given the presence of negative attentional biases, as described in Chapter 2, the patient may not notice or remember transitory positive experiences arising during mindfulness practice. Or, as a result of negative cognitive schemas (e.g., beliefs like "I'm a loser" and "I can never do anything right"), the patient might actively and consciously discount their success experiences during mindfulness practice. Here, your goal is to undo such maladaptive cognitive biases and have the person relish their success and bathe in their fundamental goodness.

> Phenomenology helps the patient to recognize, savor, and learn from therapeutic experiences.

Getting phenomenological provides a "handle" by which cognition can be grasped to help the patient to cultivate a competent use of their own mental capacities, gaining agency over thought, emotion, and body sensation (Depraz et al., 2003). Indeed, "becoming aware of lived experience is a skill that can and should be learned and practiced" (Froese et al., 2011, p. 254). During the process of phenomenological inquiry in MORE, putting one's experience into words provides a concrete way of getting a handle on one's mind (Vygotsky, 1978). Or, as Bill Miller (1983) described the importance of this process, "I learn what I believe as I hear myself talk" (p. 151). In other words, getting phenomenological helps the patient to learn from the experience of mindfulness. If the patient can express a therapeutic experience in words, and break it down into clear steps and sequences, then the patient will be more likely to be able to follow those same steps and sequences again to achieve a similar experience in the future. Furthermore, in delivering MORE as a group therapy, when a patient can get phenomenological and break down their therapeutic experience into clear steps and sequences, it is more likely that another patient will listen and be able to follow these steps to achieve a similarly therapeutic experience.

And now to the "how" of phenomenology. Bringing phenomenology into practice in MORE involves questions focused on the following:

• *Steps and sequences*—elicit descriptions of the series of events that occurred during the mind–body skill practice session. Ask, "What did you experience first? What happened next? And then what happened after that? What steps did you take to get from one state of mind (e.g., feeling stressed) to another (e.g., peace and contentment)?" Often, asking the patient to "walk me through what you just experienced" can be helpful.

• *Effect*—inquire about the effect of the various steps that occurred in the mind. "When you shifted your focus to your breath, what was the effect on your thoughts?"

• *Quality*—focus on the quality of the embodied experience as a means of enriching retrieval, obtaining more details, and further sharpening interoceptive awareness. "What did that experience feel like? What kind of sensations came up for you in that moment? Where did you feel that feeling in your body?"

• *Unusual experiences*—explore nonordinary feelings, thoughts, images, or states of consciousness. Often, patients are reluctant to talk about such experiences for fear that others will think they are "weird" or "crazy." Yet, the altered states of consciousness that arise during mindfulness practice may have powerful therapeutic implications. So, actively uncover and dig into them. "That sounds like an unusual experience. Tell me more about that."

• *Emotional tone*—focus on positive emotional experience as a means of savoring and positive rumination. Rather than let a positive experience slip by virtually unnoticed or disregarded, here you focus the patient's attention upon the feeling state evoked by that experience as a means of amplifying reward processing. "That sounds like it felt good. Tell me more about that."

- *Leading*—direct the patient to describe what was happening at different points in time throughout the experience. "So, when you got to the 'space of the sky' portion of the meditation, what happened? What happened just before and just after you had that experience?"

Central to phenomenology is the effort to "bracket" (*epoché*; Lutz & Thompson, 2003) your own theoretical explanations as a therapist, setting them aside, and then help the patient return to describe the thoughts, emotions, sensations, or state of consciousness that arose during their mind–body skill practice. In other words, to be phenomenological in one's approach involves suspending belief in what we ordinarily take for granted—one's preconceived notions of what a given experience means—and instead focusing on the raw, lived experience itself. For instance, if the patient states, "I felt relaxed," rather than assuming you understand what the word *relaxed* means, you could probe into that experience, asking questions like

> "Tell me about the exact moment when you noticed the feeling of relaxation. In that moment, what steps did you take in your mind to lead to this feeling of being relaxed? When you felt relaxed, where did you notice that feeling in your body? What did it feel like, physically in the body, and what did it feel like in terms of your emotions? Did you notice any images come to mind?"

The phenomenological approach used in MORE follows a micro-phenomenological method that allows the interviewer to obtain descriptions with a fine degree of granularity of the micro-dynamics (i.e., moment-to-moment changes) of a single experience (Depraz et al., 2003; Petitmengin et al., 2017). In MORE, this approach begins with the directed question "What did you like best about this experience?" The patient might be likely to give an overgeneralized answer, such as "I like meditating. It is relaxing." Here, the phenomenological approach is to reorient attention from this general, abstract description to a detailed account of the specific, concrete experience occurring at that particular time. To do so, each time the patient uses an abstract term, invite the patient to describe the concrete action that underlies this term. For instance, if the patient says, "It was an experience of acceptance," you can reply, "That's great! So, walk me through this acceptance. Go back to the moment when you started accepting your experience. At that moment, what did you do to accept your experience? What were you accepting?" By phrasing one's experience as an action, this implies that the patient is a conscious actor, a person with *agency* who can take similar actions in the future to bring about a similar effect. In other words, framing experience as a series of mental actions can impart a sense of self-efficacy to the patient—for example, if the patient states, "That was so relaxing," that implies the relaxation was just a fortunate and unusual happenstance, like the chance arrival of a warm, sunny day in midwinter. Getting phenomenological by saying, "What did you do that led to you feeling relaxed?" helps to reframe the relaxation as a conscious action, one the patient has power over and is capable of repeating.

When the patient expresses comments, justifications, or beliefs about their experience, gently redirect the patient back to the concrete experience they are describing. Help the patient to evoke the concrete experience by retrieving the temporal sequencing and visual, auditory, tactile, kinesthetic, interoceptive, and emotional features of that experience. Direct the patient's attention to the unfolding of the various moments in which one state of consciousness transforms into another, asking such questions as "What did you do first?"; "What happened next?"; "What happened after that?"; "When you did this, what steps did you take?"; "When you did this, what did you feel?"; "Where did you notice that feeling in your body?"; and "What makes you aware of that?" Drilling down by asking for specifics will help to deepen access to a more enriched experience for the patient.

Phenomenology is definitely the hardest part of the PURER process, because most of us have not been trained to discuss our patient's experiences in such great detail. Instead, we are trained to use our conceptual frameworks and theories to rapidly "size up" the patient's reports and fit them into Procrustean diagnostic boxes, explanatory typologies, or classification systems, so we can move efficiently through decision trees and arrive at a treatment plan or intervention. Here, in MORE, getting phenomenological *is* the intervention, which may throw you off, leading you to think, "Is this all there is to it? It can't be so simple." But although phenomenology has a simple goal, it can be difficult to implement. Many therapists become lost in their attempts to get phenomenological with a patient. When you delve into specific concrete details of the patient's experience, it is easy to "lose the trail" and get confused about the aim of your inquiry. Remember, the goal is simple: *Get the patient to focus on the details of the positive (therapeutic) experience, in a fine-grained manner.* Phenomenological inquiry often has an iterative structure; you might feel like you are going around in circles, but that's okay. With each

> Guide the patient to focus on the details of a positive experience, in a fine-grained manner.

iteration that you help the patient evoke and redescribe their experience, the level of detail, granularity, and clarity increases. When a fine-grained description of the process by which the patient achieved a therapeutic experience emerges, you have completed this piece of work and can then move to the next step in the PURER process.

Table 5.1 and the text below provide examples of a MORE therapist working in the phenomenological mode with a patient.

THERAPIST: So, what did you like best about that experience?

PATIENT: It was great. I felt calm.

THERAPIST: That's great! I'm curious, what steps did you take in your mind to calm yourself? What did you do first?

PATIENT: Well, I focused on the feeling of the air moving into my nose. But then my mind started wandering to some worries I've been having.

THERAPIST: And when you noticed that your mind started to wander, what did you do?

PATIENT: I just told myself, "No problem, it's okay that my mind is wandering." Then I focused on my breath.

THERAPIST: That's awesome that you told yourself it was okay! And then, when you focused on your breath, what happened to the worried thoughts?

PATIENT: They started getting fainter, like they were fading away, almost dissolving.

THERAPIST: Wow! And as the thoughts started to fade away, what did you notice in your body?

TABLE 5.1. An Example of Using PURER to Process a Patient's Experience during a Mindfulness Practice Session

Phenomenology	THERAPIST: It sounds like you felt you were struggling. I'm sorry that felt so difficult. But let's go back to the beginning. So, when I said you could focus your attention on your breath, what happened then?
	PATIENT: Well, I could feel the air in my nostrils, but it was only for a few seconds.
Reinforcement Education Phenomenology	THERAPIST: Wait a second! You were able to become aware of the sensation of the air in your nostrils? That's great! That awareness was a moment of mindfulness! And after you noticed the air in your nostrils, what happened in the next moment?
	PATIENT: Then my mind started jumping a mile a minute, and I was off to the races!
Reframing Education	THERAPIST: You noticed that your mind started to wander? That's also a moment of mindfulness! Mindfulness is all about noticing wherever your mind is in that moment, and then not trying to hold onto that experience or push it away, but instead, to just watch and observe your experience. So in that moment, you were practicing mindfulness!
	PATIENT: Oh, really? I thought I was doing something wrong.
Expectancy Reframing Utilization	THERAPIST: Not at all. That's perfectly normal for your mind to be jumping around like that in the beginning. But the more you practice mindfulness, the more quickly you will notice your mind has wandered, and the more easily it will become to bring your focus back to the breath. And like I said, it's okay if your mind wanders, because each time the mind wanders, and you notice where it wanders off to, and you acknowledge and accept that thought or feeling, and return your attention back to the breath, you are strengthening your mindfulness! Now, how might you use what you are learning from this experience to help yourself in future moments?
	PATIENT: Well, I guess the next time my mind wanders during mindfulness practice I can go easier on myself, and maybe stick with the practice a little longer.
Reinforcement Expectancy	THERAPIST: That's right! Great idea about practicing acceptance! I totally agree, that will really help you deepen your practice.

PATIENT: I noticed I could breathe easier. There was this feeling of calm.

THERAPIST: Where did you feel the calm in your body?

PATIENT: Right in my abdomen.

THERAPIST: What did it feel like? Can you describe it in more detail?

PATIENT: Yeah. It felt like a pleasant warmth spreading to my body, almost like there was a sun in my core shining rays of calm everywhere.

THERAPIST: That's amazing work! How could you use those rays to help yourself in the future? [Reinforcement, education, and utilization follow . . .]

If the patient struggles to converse in this phenomenological way, you could use a Socratic approach, asking leading questions to help get the patient to discuss the features of their experience that you think might be particularly important. For instance, you might say, "So, you say you felt relaxed. I'm curious, did you experience that relaxation like a warmth or tingling? Was it in your chest, or head, or somewhere else?" If all else fails, you can walk the patient through your own experience during the mind–body skill practice, getting phenomenological with yourself. Through your own self-disclosure, this might illustrate important steps and sequences of the experience and rich details that could be therapeutic for your patient—for example, in discussing savoring homework practice, you might say,

> "You could savor a campfire. When I savor campfires, I take a few moments of mindful breathing, and then focus on the beauty of the flames. I notice how the fire moves, I enjoy the scent of the fire and the crackle of the wood. Then I become aware of feeling peaceful and calm. When I do, then I turn my attention inward and focus mindfulness on that feeling of peacefulness, to deepen that sensation. Then I imagine I could absorb that peaceful feeling like water seeping into the soil."

Furthermore, phenomenology is an essential approach to helping the patient deal with the challenges that inevitably arise during mindfulness practice. By getting phenomenological, you can help the patient to learn how to successfully navigate difficult experiences, and to recognize their own capacity for dealing with challenges. In this way, phenomenology helps to reveal the patient's innate resilience and coping capacity. When a patient reports experience with a specific challenge, or makes a global, generalized statement about their capacity (e.g., "I can't do mindfulness," "Mindfulness doesn't work for me," "I struggled during this session"), your job is to become a sleuth, and hunt for the moments of success, no matter how fleeting, that occurred during the practice session. To do so, start from the beginning of the session by breaking the patient's experience down into clear steps and sequences. The text below provides examples of a MORE therapist using phenomenology to deal with a challenge.

THERAPIST: Did you experience any challenges?

PATIENT: Yeah. I just can't do mindfulness. Mindfulness doesn't work for me.

THERAPIST: I'm sorry you had a challenging time. Would you be willing to walk me through that experience? Let's start at the beginning. When I said to focus your attention on the breath, what happened?

PATIENT: Well, I became aware of my breathing.

THERAPIST: You were aware of your breathing? Wow! What did you notice about the breath?

PATIENT: It was warm. It was flowing into my nostrils.

THERAPIST: So, you really were practicing mindfulness in that moment, noticing the feeling of the breath. After you became aware of the breath, what happened next?

PATIENT: Well, then I noticed that my mind started to wander to some stressful stuff happening at work.

THERAPIST: Wow, so you were able to catch your mind starting to wander away from the breath and into some thoughts. So, you were mindful in that moment that your attention had wandered. Great work! And in the moment when you became aware of the thoughts about the stressful things at work, what did you notice in your body?

PATIENT: I noticed a tightness in my chest and neck, where I usually feel pain.

THERAPIST: So there too when you noticed the tightness, you were practicing mindfulness. You were aware of how your thoughts can affect the sensations in your body. That's a really important realization. [Next, the therapist could give some *education* and build positive *expectancy* around the patient's ability to cope with stress.]

Utilization

In contrast to phenomenology, many MORE therapists find that utilization is the easiest step in the PURER process. Our basic assumption is that whatever experience arises during mind–body skill practice (Rumi's welcome guest) has some utility in helping the patient to address their symptoms of chronic pain, emotional distress, or addictive behaviors in daily life. To prevent the patient's therapeutic experience from being ephemeral, we can employ the utilization approach to help the patient to extend and expand the therapeutic impact to other moments. Our goal with utilization is to help the patient to use whatever they have learned from the mind–body skill practice session to help themselves deal with their symptoms outside of the session in their everyday life. In other words, utilization is all about the generalization of learning. In psychology, *generalization* is the use of past learning in present situations when the conditions are similar, using generalized patterns, principles, and similarities between past and present circumstances to effectively navigate new challenges (Banich & Caccamise, 2011). This process allows us to transfer knowledge from one situation to another.

In PURER, we engage in utilization when we ask open-ended questions, like "How can you use what you learned from this experience to help yourself in future moments?" or "Based on what you just experienced, what did you learn that will be useful to you in the future?" Or, you could use more directive questions, such as "How can you use what you just learned to help you cope with [pain/distress/craving] in the future?" In either case, the goal is to help the patient to realize that the therapeutic experience that occurred in session with you has important implications for their overall psychological growth and change outside of the session.

Reframing

While the previous two PURER steps are especially useful for accentuating positive experiences, the reframing step is a primary tool for dealing with negative or challenging experiences arising during mind–body skill practice. A wide range of challenges can arise during practice. Inevitably, the mind will wander during mindfulness practice, and often it will wander to thoughts about present, past, and future stressors or concerns. Yet most patients have a preconceived notion that mindfulness involves having a laser focus on the breath, or a totally blank mind, immersed in a state of peaceful bliss. When patients hold this misconception, they typically experience frustration and disappointment, and believe they are doing mindfulness incorrectly or are not "getting it." Even worse, some patients may come to the conclusion "I can't do mindfulness. It doesn't work for me." This belief obviously may result in disengagement or dropout from MORE. Although mental states of unwavering focus, bliss, or a mind empty of thought can occur during the practice of mindfulness, these things should be regarded as benefits (or side effects) of mindfulness—not the practice of mindfulness itself. The practice of mindfulness consists of *simply being aware of what you are experiencing in any moment, and not pushing that experience away or holding on to it, but instead simply watching it from the perspective of a witness.*

> Reframing is a tool for dealing with challenging experiences arising during mind–body skill practice.

Fortunately, with the broad definition of mindfulness embraced by MORE, nearly any experience that arises during mindfulness practice can be considered evidence that the patient is engaging in the practice successfully. This notion makes sense in light of the Zen concept of *shikantaza*, translated as "just sitting" (Dogen, 2010; Leighton, 2004). In Zen, mindfulness practice is "just sitting": The moment you sit upright with full awareness of experience, you are practicing mindfulness. In *shikantaza*, there is no destination. There is nowhere to get to, and nothing else to do but remain alert and aware of experience in the moment. Thus, the simple act of awareness is mindfulness. From this perspective, awareness of anything that arises during meditation is mindfulness. That means the patient cannot *not* practice mindfulness successfully!

This notion is particularly important in delivering MORE in a group therapy context. When a patient discusses a successful experience during mind–body skill practice, and you get phenomenological and provide reinforcement, be aware that other patients in the group may not have had such a pleasant experience, and instead may have been struggling during the practice. So the moment you begin to provide reinforcement for a positive experience, you may be alienating another patient in the group. This requires a Janus-like (i.e., two-faced) approach: reinforcing the one patient for their positive practice experience while reminding the rest of the group that any experience that arises during mindfulness practice is evidence of successful engagement in the practice. This reminder comes in the form of reframing any experience that arises during a patient's mind–body skill practice as evidence of mindfulness.

Your job as a therapist is to convince the patient of this principle. To do so, you use reframing to "pull out the golden thread" in your patient's report, to find the meaning in what they are saying that directly pertains to the concept or skill you are trying to impart. Think about the best teachers who ever taught you. What does a great teacher do when they ask a question to the class, and a student gives a nonsensical answer? The teacher pulls out the piece of the answer that does make sense, or, if the answer was a non sequitur, the teacher reframes the student's statement into something related to the point the teacher is trying to make. With the reframing step of the PURER process, you are trying to emulate this approach.

For example, in response to your effort to elicit challenges, perhaps the patient states, "I don't think I was doing it right. My mind was never quiet or empty. Instead, all I could notice was my worried thoughts." You could reframe this statement by telling the patient,

> "So, in that moment, you were mindful of having worried thoughts. Good work. You were practicing mindfulness in that moment. Remember, mindfulness isn't necessarily about having an empty or quiet mind. Mindfulness is the process of being aware of what you are thinking in any moment, and not pushing those thoughts away or holding on to them but instead simply watching and observing those thoughts. You were doing it!"

Most experiences that arise can be reframed as grist for the mill of practice. Reports of mental imagery provide another example of an opportunity for reframing. It is not uncommon for patients to report experiencing imagery during mindfulness practice. For instance, if a patient reports that during the "space of the sky" portion of the mindful breathing, they envisioned being at the beach, enjoying the clouds and sunshine, you might reframe this report by stating, "So, in that moment, you were aware that the mind was creating pleasant images. That's great! Mindfulness is the practice of becoming aware of whatever the mind is experiencing in that moment, and not trying to push it away or hold on to it but just noticing what the mind is doing." An unwitting therapist might try to correct the patient and state, "Mindfulness is not the same as guided imagery. You shouldn't try to imagine anything when you are practicing mindfulness." Such therapist behavior is likely to break rapport and lead the patient toward self-condemnation or the belief "I can't do mindfulness right. Mindfulness doesn't work for me." Rather than focusing on the part of the experience that does not directly pertain to mindfulness (the content of the mental images), a skillful MORE therapist will selectively ignore this portion of the report, and instead focus on the part of the experience that does directly connect to mindfulness (the awareness of the images). Then, through the process of successive approximation, over multiple PURER processing sessions the therapist could gently steer the patient in a more fruitful direction by selectively reinforcing moments when the client was practicing mindfulness without conjuring mental images.

The aim of reframing is to transform challenges into successes, so that rather than leaving the session feeling like a failure, the patient leaves the session feeling empowered and capable. The experience of success will generate the motivation needed to stick with mindfulness practice and stay engaged in MORE.

Education and Expectancy

Many patients have little exposure to and prior experience with the mindfulness, reappraisal, and savoring skills taught in MORE. In addition, many of the experiences that occur during the practice of these mind–body skills may be unfamiliar. As such, some patients may lack the knowledge needed to understand how these experiences can help them to cope with addiction, emotional distress, and pain. Therefore, education is a key part of the PURER process. In some ways, education is the most familiar technique in the PURER process, because most clinicians are used to educating their patients about their condition and the skills they can use to address their symptoms. In other ways, education is one of the more challenging PURER steps, because to educate a client about the experiences that arise during mind–body skill practice requires intimate familiarity with these skills, as well as with mind–body theories and research discoveries. Although Chapters 2 and 3 touched on these topics, entire books (if not entire libraries!) have been written on these subjects, so spelling out everything that is known about chronic pain and addiction, as well as mindfulness, reappraisal, and savoring, is far beyond the scope of this book. Therefore, to skillfully educate the patient, a MORE therapist should actively pursue continuing education and scholarly reading on these topics (see the Appendix). Perhaps even more importantly, as mentioned in Chapter 1, a MORE therapist should have their own daily mindfulness practice. Many of the states of consciousness that arise during mindfulness meditation are so subtle or unusual that academic study alone is not sufficient: You must have the lived experience of navigating such states during mindfulness practice in order to help your patient to comprehend and troubleshoot their own practice.

To educate effectively, you need to think on your feet, responding to phenomenological reports of practice experience by informing the patient about what is happening to them, why it is happening, and/or what the experience means in terms of their health and well-being. In this way, education allows patients to grasp ahold of their practice experience and understand its significance. As the old maxim says, "Knowledge is power."

For example, during your attempt to get phenomenological, a patient might report, "It was weird. I noticed that just by watching my thoughts and feelings, they went away on their own. I didn't have to force them out of my mind." In response, you could educate them about the concept of acceptance versus resistance, saying something like

> "Yes! That's a really important insight. This is one of the things that mindfulness teaches us. You don't have to push thoughts and feelings away. In fact, research shows that when you try to suppress an unwanted thought or feeling, it often comes back even stronger! In contrast, by using mindfulness to simply watch our experiences, and accept them, without trying to get rid of them, they fade away on their own—no experience lasts forever, because in the brain the activation of neurons just comes and goes."

One kind of mindfulness experience that occurs frequently deserves a particular type of educational response. Often, patients report feelings of relaxation, calm, contentment, or peace during mindfulness practice. In a survey of over 1,000 meditation practitioners, nearly half of those sampled reported experiencing such positive emotional states "almost always" during meditation (Vieten et al., 2018). Less commonly, patients report intense feelings of joy, bliss, or even ecstasy (about one-third of the sample reported experiencing ecstasy "many times" during meditation), sometimes accompanied by the sensation of energy flowing in the body; experiences of vibration, buzzing, weightlessness or floating; or even imagery of colored lights and geometric or organic patterns behind closed eyes (Vieten et al., 2018). Although there are a number of philosophical explanations of such phenomena as described by Buddhist, Hindu, and Tantric teachers, in MORE, we often use a simple neuroscientific model to explain such phenomena. When patients report such experiences, you should educate them by saying something like

> "We know from neuroscience that when we have a really pleasurable experience like the one you just described, your brain is releasing its own opioids, called *endorphins*. Endorphins are the brain's pleasure chemical. So, when you use mindfulness [or reappraisal or savoring] to produce an experience of pleasure like that, your brain is producing its own opioids. You are creating a natural high! And if you can use your mind to release your body's own natural, healthy opioids internally, then maybe you won't need to take external opioids to feel better. You can make yourself feel better, naturally!"

This statement is particularly powerful in light of the Calvinist, Puritanical roots of modern American culture. There is much emphasis on working hard, on achievement, and on being approved by and accepted by others. In contrast, we do not typically teach our children how to make themselves feel good, naturally. Instead, there is an incessant seeking for the next and greatest achievement: If only I can obtain X, Y, and Z, then I will finally be happy. So, in MORE we educate the patient that they have the innate capacity to make themselves feel good, and we teach them concrete ways of actualizing this important capability of the human mind.

Another frequent mindfulness experience deserves special mention as a topic for education: self-transcendence. During the practice of mindfulness, sometimes patients experience brief moments in which their sense of self seems to fade away into the empty space of awareness. Other times patients might experience a sense of interconnectedness or oneness with the world or universe around them. These experiences can be disconcerting, especially when the patient has no education or context for such unusual states of mind. Yet, as previously mentioned and as we discuss in more detail in Chapter 7, self-transcendent experiences can be therapeutic. Recognize and call them out when they arise. For instance, in getting phenomenological, a patient might report something like

"I was focused intensely on my breath for several minutes. After a while, I didn't notice any thoughts or feelings. I didn't notice anything at all, not even myself! You mentioned that my mind could be like the space of the sky. It was just an open, empty space. I was awake, and aware, but I wasn't there. Am I going crazy?"

In response to such a report, you should provide education, saying something like

"Not at all! In fact, what you just described is an experience that happens every once in a while. In the ancient traditions that mindfulness comes from, this kind of experience is considered an experience of self-transcendence, in which you are connecting with something greater than yourself. The ancient mindfulness traditions considered such experiences to be a signpost that your practice is deepening. To have such a profound change in your sense of self, there have got to be changes happening in your brain. Well, we've talked about how all pain is in the brain. If pain is in the brain, and you can use mindfulness to change the way your brain functions, then you can change your pain! So, I'm curious, what was your experience of pain like in that moment?"

In this way, education could flow into another round of getting phenomenological, to help the patient to realize that cultivating self-transcendence is a way of alleviating pain.

Last, it is a useful educational practice to label the types of coping behaviors patients use in everyday life with the vocabulary of the MORE program—for example, a patient might tell you they thought about one of the stressors from their lives from an alternative perspective. You could respond, "That's great, so you were practicing reappraisal!" Or, a patient might inform you that they coped with pain by noticing the spaces inside the pain where there was no pain at all. You could respond, "Wow, so you were practicing zooming in to pain." Using the vocabulary of the MORE program will help patients to identify and become familiar with the concrete skills and practices taught in MORE, and will help connect concepts you've discussed previously with the patient's everyday experience. Similarly, you might seed the future introduction of concepts you have not discussed yet by labeling patients' spontaneous reports of these concepts. For instance, in Session 2 of MORE a patient might tell you they noticed they were able to use mindfulness to focus on and enjoy having a cup of tea in the morning. You could label that practice savoring, and tell the patient you will discuss this concept in more depth in Session 4. Using the vocabulary and concepts of MORE will help integrate the psychoeducational portions of the program with the patient's ongoing lived experience, facilitating a deeper form of learning.

The *E* in PURER also signifies expectancy. In PURER, we aim to help our patients build positive, therapeutic expectancies about the impact of mind–body skill practice. The science of expectancy is quite clear: Believing a treatment is effective actually increases its effectiveness. It doesn't matter whether the treatment is a psychological therapy, a medicine, or a surgical procedure; therapeutic expectancy powerfully shapes the outcome of that treatment. Because this phenomenon is so powerful, all rigorous clinical trials of drugs must be placebo controlled. Just believing you have received an active treatment produces symptom relief. Although therapeutic expectancies impact all forms of medical and psychological treatment, they are perhaps nowhere as powerful as in pain management. The literature on placebo and pain relief is vast. In summary, placebos can produce large effects on pain relief, by virtue of modulating various analgesic brain functions, including the release of endogenous opioids (endorphins; Colloca & Barsky, 2020; Wager et al., 2007). For instance, in a now-famous study, patients undergoing arthroscopic surgery of the knee were randomized to receive a true arthroscopic surgery, or a placebo condition in which an incision was made into the skin of the knee, but no arthroscopic procedure was completed. Patients receiving the placebo surgery showed improvements in pain and function that were equivalent to those produced by the real arthroscopic procedure (Moseley et al., 2002)! Even in open-label placebo studies, where patients are informed that they are taking a placebo, the placebo medication can produce significant pain relief (Carvalho et al., 2016). In MORE we want to maximize this expectancy effect by suggesting to the patient that the skills they are learning will help them. In addition to direct statements to this effect, you can tell the patient, "Research has shown that mindfulness reduces pain and addictive behavior while improving well-being." You might cite specific results from a specific study to hammer home this point. For instance, you could discuss the results from my good colleague Fadel Zeidan and his team (Zeidan et al., 2011, 2015), who experimentally induced pain by placing a hot metal probe on participants' legs, and found that mindfulness practice significantly reduced pain intensity while altering analgesic responses in the brain. You could discuss the results from the largest clinical trial of MORE, stating that patients were continuing to experience pain relief 9 months after the end of the 8-week treatment, and patients were able to significantly reduce their opioid use for the long-term (Garland, Hanley, Nakamura, et al., 2022). Alternatively, you could talk about a former patient whom you (or one of your colleagues) treated who experienced relief from MORE.

The same tactic can be used to build positive expectancy around developing mindfulness, reappraisal, and savoring skills. Suggesting "the more you practice, the better you will get at [mindfulness/reappraisal/savoring]," will build the motivation to engage in mind–body skill practice in spite of the inevitable challenges that arise—for example, when patients report experiencing mind wandering during mindfulness meditation, you could provide education to normalize this challenge as part of the learning process, and then build expectancy by reassuring the patient, "Each time you practice mindfulness, you will catch your mind wandering more quickly, and it will become easier to let those wandering thoughts go. Eventually, you will find that your mind wanders less and less, and the spaces in between thoughts will grow larger and longer."

Reinforcement

Positive reinforcement is the essence of PURER. Although it is represented as the last letter in the PURER acronym, you should use reinforcement early on and liberally in processing. Essentially, you should reinforce any patient report that even slightly indicates that a therapeutic experience has occurred. And recall *shikantaza*—at minimum, the patient was "just sitting" with their experience, and should at minimum be positively reinforced for attending to their present-moment experience with full awareness, regardless of the content of their experience. Remember that many patients are suffering from a deep-seated sense of worthlessness, self-hatred, hopelessness, and depression. Receiving authentic positive reinforcement from a therapist can be powerfully healing for transforming one's self-image. And of course, over 100 years of behavioral research has clearly demonstrated that positive reinforcement is one of the most powerful means of facilitating the learning and acquisition of novel (adaptive) behaviors.

> Use reinforcement early on and liberally.

In MORE, we provide positive reinforcement by communicating affirmation, support, and encouragement to our patients through kind words and gestures (a high five, a handshake coupled with a smile). Authenticity and enthusiasm are significant here. Phrases like "Good job!"; "Great work!"; "You're really getting it!"; and "That's amazing!" carry weight when you point to the specifics of what the patient has done. For instance, effective reinforcement is exemplified by the statement "Great work! I'm amazed at how you've been able to use mindfulness to cope with feelings of anger." Authenticity in reinforcement arises naturally out of awareness that it really is amazing when a patient suffering from complex intersecting comorbidities like physical pain, trauma, depression, and opioid misuse can mindfully focus on the breath to experience a moment of relief amid all of their anguish. It takes hard work to learn mind–body skills in the face of such extreme life adversity. The patient's hard work should be acknowledged by genuine words of affirmation, which will help motivate them to continue with the practice, in spite of difficulty. Positive reinforcement is a strong antidote to the crippling self-doubt and lack of self-efficacy that are ubiquitous in the clinical populations to be treated by MORE.

Finally, positive reinforcement can be combined with building expectancy. For instance, if a patient has a therapeutic experience in the first couple of sessions, you could state,

> "Wow! That's amazing that you had that experience. What that tells me is there is a really good prognosis for mindfulness being able to help you. If you got this much benefit already in our first session, by the eighth session, I can't even imagine how much better you are going to feel! Mindfulness is really going to work for you!"

Messages like this can be powerfully reinforcing.

When and How to Use PURER

To be clear, PURER is a guiding framework for helping the patient to process their mind–body skill experience. However, PURER is heuristic rather than prescriptive—it is meant to guide and inform your inquiry with the patient, but not to dictate exactly what you say and how you say it. You do not have to go through each PURER step with every patient; indeed, for most group MORE sessions, you will not have enough time to go through each PURER step with each patient. You will likely only have time to do the PURER process with what three patients "liked best," and perhaps with one or two challenges. In order to ensure you are treating each patient with the PURER process, it can be helpful to elicit responses from different patients in every session. In this way, not every patient has the opportunity to go through PURER in every session, but will have the opportunity to do so within two or three sessions.

Also, you do not need to follow the PURER steps in the order specified in the acronym. For instance, for some patient reports, the most immediately appropriate step to take is reinforcement, whereas for other patient reports, you should begin by providing education, or getting phenomenological. By and large, starting with phenomenology is often the best approach. Nonetheless, you should tailor your response to the participant comment or report, rather than following the PURER approach in a sequential fashion. Often, the process becomes quite circular and iterative—for example, beginning with phenomenology, then moving to reframing, followed by education, and then returning to phenomenology before finishing with utilization and reinforcement. With each iteration of phenomenology, the patient may become better able to describe their experience with greater clarity, leading to a deeper and more generalizable form of learning—the goal of the PURER process. See Table 5.1 for some examples of therapist–patient dialogue as related to the PURER steps.

When to Ask about Relief

When in the PURER process should you inquire about symptom relief? After 15 years of studies on MORE, and listening to countless hours of audio recordings of MORE therapists working with patients, I have discovered that there is indeed an optimal time to ask about relief. In getting phenomenological, when the patient reports experiencing some sort of positive mental state (e.g., pleasant thoughts, emotions, body sensations, or states of consciousness), after you've explored that mental state and helped the patient to enrich their description of the positive state, that is the ideal moment to inquire about symptom relief. The logic here is simple: Pleasant and unpleasant experiences lie at opposite ends of the hedonic continuum. It is difficult (though perhaps not impossible) to feel good and bad at the same time. When a patient reports feeling relaxed, content, peaceful, joyful, or even bliss during a mindfulness practice session, it is highly unlikely that in that particular moment they were also suffering anguish from symptoms of physical pain, emotional pain, or craving. Pain and craving may have been present, but it is not likely these symptoms were particularly bothersome, in the context of the positive affective states just noted. During that particular state in that particular moment, it is likely that the patient was experiencing relief—thus, you are stacking the deck in your favor by asking about symptom relief at that moment. Per our discussion of the anatomy of a mindfulness meditation in Chapter 4, the way you ask the question makes all the difference. If you ask a closed question, "Did mindfulness make your pain better?," you are likely to get a response of "No way—I'm always in pain." Contrary responses like that are due to a kind of resistance. From the perspective of motivational interviewing (Miller & Rollnick, 2023), resistance is what happens when we expect or push for change when the patient is not ready for that change. So instead of pushing the patient by implying that mindfulness will relieve their pain, you could state, "So you said that during mindfulness you experienced this sense of relaxation and peace. You described it as an enveloping warmth that spread from your heart all throughout your torso, even to your back. I'm just curious, in that moment, what was your experience of pain like?" Time and time again, I have heard patients in MORE sessions respond to this question by saying, "Pain? Oh yeah, my pain. Now that you mention it, I didn't really notice my pain very much in that moment, maybe not even at all." A skillful response to this description would be something like "Wow! In that moment, you didn't really notice your pain. Your pain was temporarily gone. So, it sounds like one of the things you might be realizing is that mindfulness is a way to alleviate your pain, naturally!" The same type of approach could be used to help the patient to recognize relief of emotional distress, or craving for opioids, resulting from mind–body skill practice.

By concluding the first five chapters of this book, you now have a solid grasp of the problem of chronic pain and opioid misuse, the theoretical framework underlying MORE, the strategy behind MORE's approach to teaching mindfulness, and how to motivate learning and growth through the PURER process. In Chapter 6, I outline details on delivering the MORE treatment sessions.

Chapter 6

Notes on Delivering the Sessions

In the chapters that follow, the eight sessions of MORE are detailed. These sessions closely follow the MORE treatment manual that we have tested, optimized, and refined over the past 15 years across multiple clinical trials. Each session is complete with an agenda, an approximate time duration for each activity, notes to the therapist outlining the focus of the session and pitfalls to be avoided, a script to be read to patients, discussion questions, and mind–body exercises. You may read the session script word for word to your patients, or you can view the session script as a general guideline of themes to discuss with your patients. Once you learn the material well you can deliver it in your own words, with your own metaphors. That said, it is strongly recommended that you read the text of the guided mindfulness meditations and other mind–body practices word for word, at least until you come to a deep understanding of each practice and the suggestions that are embedded therein. The language and sequencing of suggestions in these techniques are designed specifically to activate therapeutic mechanisms integral to the MORE treatment approach (as described in Chapter 3). If you significantly modify wording of these guided practices, they may lose some of their efficacy.

Points to Consider before Embarking on Delivering MORE

Session Structure and Temporal Orientation

MORE is a complex intervention with many moving parts. Each session involves mindfulness meditation, in-depth processing through the PURER approach, psychoeducation with discussion questions, additional mind–body techniques (e.g., reappraisal, savoring), and assignment of home practice. To deliver all this content within the typical 2-hour timeframe requires a therapist to be highly structured. You will need to keep the session tightly focused on the topics at hand, and not allow for much extraneous conversation. This approach is different from the typical therapy session, where the patient usually details the psychological experiences and stressors that occurred after the last treatment session or describes earlier life experiences and traumas. By way of contrast, in MORE, therapy should be largely focused on the patient's present-moment experience (e.g.,

> Keep the session tightly focused on the topics at hand.

phenomenological exploration of thoughts and feelings that arise during meditation) with an eye toward how the patient can attain their therapeutic goals (e.g., reduce their opioid use) and achieve psychological growth.

Processing of Mind–Body Practice

As a reminder, you will be processing mindfulness and other mind–body practices, as well as the home practice of these techniques, using the PURER approach. However, as discussed in Chapter 5, you will not have enough time to be able to do the PURER process with each patient for every mind–body practice. You will probably have enough time to process with two to three patients for each mind–body practice in the session. Therefore, you should process each mind–body practice with different patients across different sessions. By spreading your attention around the group in this way, you will implement the PURER process with each patient over the course of a few sessions.

Addiction Content

If you are not working with patients with opioid misuse and OUD, you should omit the content around addiction as it is not relevant to patients who have not progressed to that stage of opioid use, and instead keep the sessions focused on relieving chronic pain and reducing opioid dosing if it is medically appropriate and consistent with the patients' goals. If you are working with a mixed group comprising patients who take opioids as prescribed for chronic pain as well as those who misuse opioids, those who are actively addicted to opioids, and/or those receiving treatment for OUD (e.g., methadone or buprenorphine), you should present the addiction-related content in the sessions. In this case, at the beginning of the session inform the participants that you will be discussing topics that may not match the symptoms of every group member. Nonetheless, that information could still be useful for them. You could say something like the following:

> "I know that not everyone misuses opioids or has an addiction. If I bring up a topic related to opioid misuse or addiction, and it doesn't directly apply to you, you still might learn something from the discussion that could be useful in preventing future problems for yourself or others."

> Spread your attention around the group over a few sessions to cover PURER with each patient.

Gradual Motivational Approach toward Changing Opioid Use

In MORE, we aim to meet the patient "where they are" in terms of their motivation to change. Often this means starting by teaching the patient to use mindfulness to alleviate pain, rather than to change their opioid use. For patients who are still in the precontemplation stage of change, directives to reduce (or quit) opioid use will likely be met with resistance. Rather than directly confronting patients about their opioid use, we first ask them to bring mindfulness to their opioid use patterns through the STOP technique—a practice of cultivating awareness in the moments before taking opioids (see Session 1). As the sessions unfold, you should gradually draw more and more attention to the patient's opioid use, using PURER processing to help the patient to discriminate between the motivation to take opioids to obtain pain relief versus other motivations indicative of opioid misuse (e.g., the desire to alleviate negative emotional states). In Session 5, you will introduce the concept of craving and encourage patients to consider whether craving is a factor in motivating their opioid use. Often, this is a key moment that leads the patient to move to readiness to change their opioid use patterns. As some patients in the group begin to report increasing the time between their opioid doses, or skipping doses, provide ample reinforcement of these changes and build positive expectancy that they can continue to reduce their dose and potentially even taper off of opioids entirely if that is their goal.

Having such discussions will provide valuable modeling for other patients in the group who have not yet begun to change their dose patterns. As always, perform the "Janus-faced" maneuver of reinforcing the patient who is successfully reducing their dose while expressing acceptance toward the other patients who are not yet ready to make that change (e.g., "Now

> Recognizing how craving operates is a key moment that leads the patient to move to readiness to change.

I know that everyone is an individual and there's no one right opioid dose for everyone. Only you can know when the right moment is to change your opioid use").

Addressing Relapse

Relapse is common among patients with OUD who are trying to abstain from drug use and among those who are in addiction treatment. If, during a MORE session, a patient reports a drug use episode in the previous week, you should use PURER to help them to unpack what happened in the moments leading up to, during, and after the drug use. Get *phenomenological* and help the patient recognize what triggered the drug use. Help them to become aware of whether their drug use was a conscious choice or the result of activation of an automatic habit. Reduce shame by providing *education* about relapse and normalizing drug use as part of addiction recovery. *Reframe* the lapse as an opportunity to learn how to use the MORE skills to strengthen recovery. Then, ask

> Reframe the lapse as an opportunity to learn how to use the MORE skills to strengthen recovery.

the patient how they attempted to *utilize* mindfulness, reappraisal, and/or savoring skills to manage their cravings and drug use in the situation. If they did not attempt to use the MORE skills, describe how they could use mindfulness, reappraisal, and savoring in the future to reduce the urge to use drugs and/or moderate their use. Walk the patient through the use of these skills or have another patient in the group describe how they used such skills successfully in the past to reduce craving and prevent a relapse. Finally, provide *reinforcement* to the patient for continuing the MORE treatment and remaining dedicated to recovery, and build positive *expectancy* that with practice, they will become better able to use the skills they have learned to manage the urge to use drugs and prevent relapse.

Patient Comfort and Breaks

You should be aware that when working with chronic pain, sometimes patients will need to get up from their chairs, stretch, stand, or move around. They might also need to lie down on the floor.

When you set the ground rules for the sessions during Session 1, you should give patients explicit permission to adjust their body posture as necessary to enable them to stay engaged for the entire length of the treatment session. That said, there can also be benefit in learning to practice mindfulness through an experience of discomfort. Practicing mindfulness to tolerate the discomfort of an itch, the desire to fidget, or a backache can be a powerful learning experience. On a related note, a standard 2-hour MORE group format includes a 10-minute break approximately halfway through the session, to allow patients to move as needed, get food or drink, take a bathroom break, and so on.

Guided Home Practice

When learning mindfulness and other mind–body practices, guided home practice is very useful. Although there are innumerable meditation apps and guided meditations available on the internet, the wording of the mind–body practices in MORE is very specific and designed to modulate particular mechanisms as described in Chapter 3. Furthermore, your patients have developed a therapeutic relationship and rapport with you, and as such, they have connected with *your voice*. Thus, from the principle of synchrony (as described in Chapter 4), patients will go more deeply into the state of mindfulness when they practice along with a recording of your voice, as opposed to the voice of a stranger. In that regard, your patients should have audio recordings of you guiding them through each of the major mind–body practices in MORE. You could record yourself delivering each of the practices and distribute this recording to your patients, or you could allow your patients to record your voice as you deliver the practices in each of the sessions. Most smartphones have a "voice recorder" app that can be used to produce a decent quality recording of your voice as you deliver each mind–body practice. These recordings can then be emailed to your patients, who can then play the recording with their smartphone when they are ready to practice.

Home Practice Noncompliance

If participants do not complete their home practice (this is a not uncommon occurrence), you should adopt a simple behavioral approach. Ask the patient to describe their daily schedule, and help them identify times of the day when they can practice. Then ask the patient whether they can commit to practicing at this day and time, and tell them you will follow up in the next session to make sure that this practice time worked for them. Discussing the benefits of, and barriers to, practice can also help increase patient motivation to practice. The more mind–body practice the participant engages in, the more likely they are to benefit from MORE. That said, some patients never practice at home outside of the MORE sessions, so you should make the in-session mindfulness practice highly impactful. Hence, the tools and tactics discussed in Chapters 4 and 5 are essential.

Supplemental Session on Self-Transcendence in Recovery

MORE has continued to evolve over the years as informed by key discoveries from our research. For nearly a decade we

> The more mind–body practice the participant engages in, the more likely they are to benefit from MORE.

heard reports from MORE patients and therapists that self-transcendent experiences do occur with some frequency during mind–body practices over the course of the 8-week intervention. We then embarked upon the scientific investigation of these experiences and found evidence of the clinical importance of self-transcendence as a therapeutic mechanism of MORE (Garland, Hanley, Hudak, et al., 2022; Garland, Hanley, Riquino, et al., 2019; Hanley & Garland, 2022; Hudak et al., 2021). Consequently, some therapists are interested in providing psychoeducation and meditation practices to point more directly to self-transcendence throughout the intervention. If you feel that such a focus is appropriate and might be helpful for your patient, you may use the material described in Chapter 7 as a supplemental session on the role of self-transcendence in recovery from chronic pain, opioid misuse, and OUD. I recommend that you deliver this material after Session 7 and before the final session on "Maintaining Mindful Recovery" in Session 8. Note that unlike the eight sessions in this book, the supplemental material in Chapter 7 has not been fully vetted in randomized controlled trials (RCTs). Although this material should be considered experimental based on our scientific work in this area, I have every reason to believe that focusing on self-transcendence may facilitate recovery enhancement and psychological growth in many patients treated with MORE.

With these considerations in mind, now, on to the sessions!

The MORE Sessions

Session 1

Mindfulness of Physical and Emotional Pain

Agenda

Set ground rules regarding confidentiality and group discussion: 10 minutes

Introductions: 10 minutes

The purpose of the program: 5 minutes

The nature of pain: 20 minutes

Introduction to mindfulness: 15 minutes

Break: 10 minutes

Body scan practice: 10 minutes

Process body scan (using PURER): 10 minutes

Coping with pain by zooming in: 5 minutes

Mindful breathing practice: 10 minutes

Process mindful breathing practice (using PURER): 5 minutes

Assignment for home practice: 10 minutes—discuss and assign for the following week:

- Daily mindful breathing or body scan practice
- STOP practice

Materials Needed

Handout S1.1. What Is Pain and Why Can Mindfulness Help?

Handout S1.2. The Loop of Mindfulness

Handout S1.3. Zooming in to Pain

Handout S1.4. Mindfulness Practice

Handout S1.5. STOP Practice

Session Introduction for the Therapist

This session provides a rationale for mindfulness as a solution for chronic pain. Mindfulness is the first and most central pillar of the MORE approach. Presenting this rationale is critical for helping patients develop a positive expectancy for the therapeutic effects of MORE. Unlike the other seven sessions, this session is heavily focused on psychoeducation. The session introduces the first mindfulness technique, a body scan, intended to help increase awareness that pain is composed of sensory, cognitive, and emotional factors. Be cognizant that this first body scan may not relieve pain, so do not set the expectation for pain relief with this initial practice. The intention of the body scan in Session 1 is simply to illustrate the construct of mindfulness. Then the session ends by introducing the core practice of mindful breathing that is expanded upon in later sessions as the primary pain-relieving technique taught in MORE.

Therapist Notes

When you introduce yourself, make sure you describe how you came to mindfulness and how your own practice of mindfulness has benefited your life. This personal testimonial increases your credibility, sets a precedent for disclosing deeply held feelings and beliefs, and sets an expectation for the positive effects of mindfulness practice. After you introduce yourself, set ground rules for the group and expectations for confidentiality, as is appropriate for your treatment setting.

Watch the time here and do not allow introductions to go beyond 10 minutes, as patients otherwise may tell long emotional stories that can use up valuable time needed to deliver the psychoeducation and mindfulness techniques in this session. Concise, but pointed, emotional disclosure is best. After you have completed the introductions, the focus of this first session shifts to you providing the group members with some psychoeducational background to help them understand what MORE is all about, the nature of pain, and how mindfulness can help. You also introduce the group to the fundamental mindfulness practices: body scan and mindful breathing.

Session Script

Text that is **_boldfaced and italicized_** here and throughout these eight sessions is intended to provide suggested discussion questions to raise with the group members.

Introductions

Let's take some time to go around and introduce ourselves. Take a minute and tell us about yourself. Can you tell us about your experience with chronic pain and opioids? How do you hope these sessions will help you with chronic pain? What do you hope to get out of this experience?

Purpose of the MORE Program

Welcome to the Mindfulness-Oriented Recovery Enhancement (MORE) program. The purpose of this eight-session program is to give you skills and tools for reducing pain, stress, and opioid use. These sessions offer different things for different people. Some people want to learn psychological skills to add to their traditional pain management strategies to get even more pain relief and improve their quality of life. Some people are happy with the dose of opioid medication they are taking. Other people want to use the skills in these sessions to help them use less opioid medication to manage their condition. Others want to try to get off opioid medication entirely by learning to use the skills in these sessions as their primary pain management approach. If you are addicted to opioids, you may be interested in reducing your opioid use or breaking free from your addiction. If you are being treated with medications for opioid use disorder (OUD), you may be trying to stay off of drugs and strengthen your recovery, but you might also be interested in learning to manage your pain. In fact, approximately 50% of those who developed an OUD started using opioids for pain relief. Some people use opioids to not only alleviate physical pain but also to manage emotional pain, like stress, depression, anxiety, anger, shame, and resentment. And this program could be useful in providing an alternative way of coping with difficult emotions. It's good that there are many different types of people in this group. We can all learn from one another.

I want to be clear that we will not tell you to decrease your opioid medication use during this program—that's a choice that only you can make in collaboration with your doctor. Cutting down your opioid medication is a serious thing that should be managed by your doctor. During this 8-week program, if you wish to reduce your prescribed dose of medication, you should consult with your doctor about how you should go about doing this. If you want to decrease your dose, and your doctor thinks it is appropriate, I fully support and encourage you to reduce your medication. To be clear, sometimes it doesn't make sense to decrease your use of opioid medication. For example, if you are taking medications for OUD, stopping taking those medications might lead to a relapse. On the other hand, in some situations, decreasing use of opioid analgesics like oxycodone or hydrocodone can often improve your health.

This program is not the same thing as a support group. Support is important, and I hope that you find support from one another in this group. However, this program offers more than support: It offers practical techniques so that you can learn to help yourself. To get the most out of this program, it requires practice not only during our meetings but also practice during the rest of the week. At the end of every meeting, we will go over a few home practice assignments for the next week. The more practice you do at home, the better you will learn the skills, and the more improvement you will experience. Some of the things we talk about in this program will be familiar; others will be totally new, and might even sound weird. That's okay. If you have any questions about anything in the program, please ask them. Also, your participation in this program is totally voluntary. You do not have to do any of the activities you don't want to do. However, other people around you will be interested in learning, so please be respectful of that. Many of the activities we will do in the program will involve silent reflection and quiet focus, so please be respectful of your neighbor and don't talk while others are trying to be quiet. There will be ample time to ask questions and give your opinion throughout each program meeting. Lastly, I'm going to ask you questions about your experience with the skills that I teach you. I'm not asking these questions to pick on you, or to be nosy, or rude. I'm asking them to get a clear understanding of what you are experiencing, so I can be a good coach and help you use the skills more effectively.

In this program, we will be spending time talking about pain and the use of opioid medication, like oxycodone, hydrocodone, and methadone. There is a lot of stigma in our society around opioid use.

Have you ever felt stigmatized by your use of opioids?

There is also a lot of stigma in our society around the emotional aspects of pain. For instance, some people fear that if they admit there are emotional aspects to their pain, others will think their pain is "all in their head."

Have you ever felt stigmatized about the emotional aspects of your pain?

Before we proceed, I want to be clear about the philosophy behind this program with regard to opioid use and the emotional aspects of pain. MORE is founded on the idea that people are doing the best they can do to cope with the challenges in life at that moment. If someone is using opioids, they are using opioids because they feel that they need opioids to cope in that moment. There is nothing morally "wrong" about that. Even if a person takes more opioids than prescribed, or in a different way than prescribed (such as taking opioids with alcohol or weed, or taking opioids to relieve stress and emotional suffering), there is nothing morally "wrong" about that. From the perspective of MORE, people do what they need to do to cope. Period. This isn't a moral issue. It may be a health issue, however, in that certain types of coping may be more or less effective and more or less hurtful to the body and mind. So, the purpose of this program is not to judge you but rather to help you to figure out "Is what I am doing working for me? And, if not, how can I do things differently?"

So let's begin by discussing how emotions and thoughts interact with the body during the experience of pain.

The Nature of Pain

Pain is actually a lot more complicated than it seems. The experience most of us call "pain" actually comprises four separate elements:

• **Nociception**, the "damage signal," sends information to the brain that the body has been damaged or is about to be damaged. That message is transmitted along nerves, from the tissue that has been damaged to the brain. If your finger gets poked by a pin, or you accidentally touch a hot burner on your stove, the nerves in your finger send a nociceptive signal up your spinal cord to tell your brain that the finger has been hurt. You don't have to be conscious of nociception for it to occur; damage could be happening to your body and you might not even be aware of it.

• **Pain**, here, refers to an uncomfortable feeling that is often associated with some kind of actual or potential damage to the body. Unlike nociception, pain is a conscious experience: It occurs within your awareness. The function of pain is to protect us: It tells you to avoid the thing that is causing the pain. For example, if you sense heat from the burner on your stove, and pull your hand back, you might feel pain, but that pain does not necessarily mean your finger has been harmed. The pain may be telling you that if you don't pay closer attention when cooking, you may do real damage to your finger.

• **Suffering** consists of the negative thoughts and emotions people have about their pain. We suffer when we get upset about our pain, when we say, "Why me? This pain is ruining my life!" or when we think "I can't handle this pain! There's nothing I can do to cope with this!" We also suffer when we judge and interpret the sensations in our body as terrible, awful, and anguishing, and when we worry about whether the pain will ever get better.

• **Reaction** is the behavior that happens when you are in pain, and what you do to cope with pain. Examples of pain reactions include groaning and wincing, scanning your attention around your body looking for other painful sensations, avoiding physical activity, staying in bed, avoiding work and social activities, reading medical websites trying to find a solution to the pain, seeking out medical treatments, drinking alcohol to numb the pain, taking opioids, and so on.

Chronic pain frequently begins after a person experiences an injury or certain kinds of diseases. Sometimes pain becomes chronic because the injured tissue in the body doesn't heal correctly, or because the nerves in that part of the body have been damaged. But sometimes pain persists even when the original injury or disease has healed. Sometimes, pain can begin to spread to parts of the body that were never injured in the first place. For some people, doctors can easily identify the source of their pain with an MRI or an X-ray, but other people who suffer from chronic pain often find that medical tests cannot identify causes for their pain.

Sometimes when someone has lived with pain for a long time, the nervous system begins to develop a habit of feeling pain. This changes the way the pain signals are processed in the brain. Pain can become "stuck in the brain" long after the injury or damage to the body has healed. In this way pain can become a memory pattern in the brain that keeps coming back even though your body is healing. This kind of chronic pain is not uncommon. People often think their chronic pain comes from an old injury, but in some cases, that injury may have healed, and yet the pain persists.

So in this way, pain and nociception are not the same thing. There can actually be pain without nociception. For example, in phantom limb pain an amputee feels pain in a hand or foot that has been cut off in an amputation. The hand is gone, but people still feel pain in the fingers of that hand. The brain creates a representation of the hand and projects the experience of pain there. Without a hand, there can be no signal of damage coming from the fingers. But, the pain is very real, as it is in some other pain conditions where no tissue damage can be found.

There can also be nociception without pain. For example, take this case report from the medical literature. A construction worker went to the dentist for a mild toothache. When he got an X-ray, the dentist discovered that a 4-inch nail had pierced through his lower jaw and cheekbone and gone up into his skull! Then the construction worker remembered that he accidentally shot himself in the head with a nail gun. After 6 days with this nail in his head, his "toothache" was bothering him enough to go the dentist and get it checked out. There was massive damage to the body, but very little pain. There are also stories of football players who break their leg and are so focused on the game that they can run on that broken leg and score a touchdown. There are stories of soldiers who get shot in war but who continue to fight in spite of the serious wound because their adrenaline is pumping and they don't feel the pain.

Have you ever had the experience of being so focused on what you are doing that you don't notice your pain?

These experiences can be explained by the way the brain processes nociception and turns it into pain. See Handout S1.1. There's a part of the brain called the thalamus that acts like a "gate" to allow the damage signal to pass up from the body into the higher, thinking part of the brain, called the prefrontal cortex [**Therapist note**: Point to your forehead.] and the sensory and emotional parts of the brain [**Therapist note**: Point above your ear.] where the damage signal is interpreted as pain. You can think of the thalamus like the volume control on an audio device. When you change the focus of your attention, your prefrontal cortex can actually open up or close down the "gate" of the thalamus, which can increase or decrease the volume (or intensity) of the pain itself. For example, the construction worker we just talked about wasn't paying attention to the fact that he had shot himself with the nail gun, so his pain gate was tightly closed and he didn't feel much pain at all. On the other hand, when people focus on their pain and start to worry about it, it can actually open the pain gate and turn up the volume of the pain. Your emotions can also influence how nociception is processed in the brain. When you are upset with emotions like anger, sadness, or fear, limbic brain structures like the amygdala can actually turn the volume of the pain up. On the other hand, when you are feeling happy, relaxed, or enjoying something pleasurable, structures in the brain's reward system (called the striatum) can turn the volume of the pain down.

Have you ever noticed when you are feeling happy or doing something that you really enjoy, that your pain doesn't bother you as much?

So, if you really think about it, pain is neither only physical nor only mental. It is both. It doesn't matter whether the pain is coming from touching a hot burner, a pin poking your finger, a nail sticking in your foot, a knot in your back, a herniated disk, an irritable bowel, or a pounding headache—the pain you experience has both physical and mental parts. Saying, "Your pain is all in your head," is nonsense—it's also unhelpful and insulting. Anytime there is pain, the person is experiencing that pain with their brain. The brain is interpreting the signals carried by the nerves from the body. And, the brain is an organ in the body, like the heart or lungs. So pain is in the body—it's physical. But anytime someone experiences a painful injury or a disease, they will have thoughts and emotions about it. In this way, pain is also happening in the mind. Often when we are in pain, we experience negative thoughts and emotions about the pain. For example, you might feel worried about whether your pain is ever going to go away, you might feel anger and resentment about how the pain has affected your day-to-day living, or you might be sad because of the losses you've experienced due to pain ("I can't hike any more" or "I can't lift heavy things anymore so I'm no longer a strong adult"). These kinds of emotional suffering can actually turn up the volume of the pain in your brain and make pain hurt worse.

When a person has experienced serious chronic pain, sometimes their pain involves negative *thoughts* like "I can't stand this pain," "There's nothing I can do to make this better," and "What if the pain never ends?" This kind of negative thinking about pain can also make pain worse, by increasing negative emotions. For example, if you have chronic back pain and you stand on your feet for an hour, your back might start to hurt. You might then think to yourself, "I'm such a wimp. I can't even stand up straight without my back hurting." These thoughts might lead you to feel shame and anger toward yourself. Then you might get tense, which would increase the tightness and aching in your back. Resentment about the injury, worry about being disabled, or feeling depressed about your limitations can aggravate the experience of pain much worse by creating suffering. And some people take opioids to help deal with these negative thoughts and emotions. While it is unfortunately true in some cases that the original injury or disease may not be very controllable, you can reduce your suffering. A wise sage (the Buddha) once likened pain and suffering to getting hit by two arrows in the exact same spot: The first arrow is the original painful condition, but the second arrow is the emotional and mental suffering that we lay on top of the pain, which makes it hurt worse.

Because pain is both physical and mental, it often requires both physical and mental therapies. I think you are familiar with physical pain therapies. You've probably tried a lot of them already: physical therapy, exercise, chiropractic, massage, pain medication, injections, and surgeries. However, these therapies do not focus on changing the way the brain processes pain, nor do they treat the negative thoughts and emotions that maintain pain and make it worse. The MORE program is focused on a therapy that not only changes the way pain is processed in the brain but also changes the mental aspects of pain and reduces suffering. This therapeutic approach involves a kind of mental training called mindfulness.

Introduction to Mindfulness

Mindfulness is a kind of training designed to exercise and strengthen your mind and brain. By training your mind, your mindfulness will become stronger. Strengthening your mindfulness can help reduce your pain and improve your quality of life. Mindfulness can also make you a happier person in general. You can think of mindfulness almost like a kind of weight lifting for your prefrontal cortex, the part of your brain involved in self-control. Here's a simple definition of mindfulness: *Mindfulness is the practice of focusing on what is happening in the present moment, right here and right now.* When you practice mindfulness, you are not getting lost in memories about the past, and you are not daydreaming about the future. Instead, you focus on what you are seeing, hearing, feeling, and thinking right now, in this moment. What is happening right now, in this moment, is that you are sitting and listening to me explain how you can use mindfulness to help yourself with chronic pain.

But that's not all. There is another important part of mindfulness. Mindfulness is the practice of focusing on what is happening in the present moment, *without judging or reacting to it, but instead just watching your experience, from the perspective of an observer or a witness.* This mode of experience is pretty different from what we typically do. Usually, we make judgments all day long about the things that happen in our life. When something happens, we usually ask ourselves, "Do I like it? Do I dislike it? Is what's happening good, or bad?" You might be judging what I'm saying to you right now. "Does it make sense, or is this a bunch of mumbo jumbo?" Our minds were designed by evolution to evaluate the events in our lives and figure out what they mean for our well-being and survival. Making judgments about the events of our lives can be really helpful. But sometimes our judgments can become hurtful. We might judge ourselves or others too harshly. We might place false blame, or come to false conclusions about the situations in our lives. Instead of coming to rash (and faulty) judgments, mindfulness is a completely different approach to use your mind. When we are mindful, we become aware of what is happening in the present moment, without judgment, without labeling the situation as good or bad, but instead, just taking it in. Just watching, just observing your experience, like an objective witness—a witness who is withholding any judgment, just taking in all the available information, staying open and attentive to anything new that might come up. When you learn how to use mindfulness to suspend your judgment and stay open, you become less reactive to what is happening in the present moment.

Do you know what I mean when I use this word *reactive*? When I am having a bad day and am really reactive, and then somebody yells at me, I yell back at them. That instinct to retaliate—that's a reaction. Or for example, let's say you get bitten by two dogs in the same week when you were walking down the street in your neighborhood. Then, the next time you walk down that street and see a dog, you are going to judge it as "bad," and then become reactive—you'll be afraid, you'll keep your eyes on the dog, you'll watch your back, or maybe even take off running away down the street! But mindfulness is all about being nonreactive. It's about seeing the dog as a new dog—and not assuming it is going to bite you just because there are a couple of poorly trained dogs on your street.

It's not uncommon to become reactive to pain. If you've experienced severe pain or medical issues in the past, and then a new pain pops up in your body, you might react by thinking the pain is a sign that something is seriously wrong with your body, that you have a disease. Or, you might react by thinking the pain is never going away and will last forever. You might even react by assuming there is nothing you can do to make your pain better—there's no way to cope with it. These kinds of reactions can make pain hurt even worse, by turning up the volume of the pain in the brain. But pain might not be a signal of a serious health problem. It might not last forever. Sometimes, chronic pain can heal on its own, given enough time. Maybe you've heard the expression

"Time heals all wounds." Some people who have lived with chronic pain for many years discover much to their surprise that their pain has healed gradually over time, bit by bit, until one day the pain no longer bothers them anymore.

In contrast to these pain reactions, mindfulness can help you to turn down the volume of your pain. Science shows that mindfulness can actually decrease the intensity of pain. In several different research studies, scientists took a metal probe, heated to about 120°F, hot enough to cause a serious burning pain, and touched it to people's legs while they practiced mindfulness meditation in a brain scanner. Mindfulness significantly reduced the intensity of the pain caused by the hot metal probe, and this decrease in pain intensity was linked with decreased activation in the thalamus, the brain's pain gate. So mindfulness turned down the volume of the pain by closing the pain gate. Science actually knows a lot about how mindfulness can decrease pain. In large studies involving many hundreds of people with all sorts of painful medical conditions, mindfulness reduces pain on average by about 30%. That's about as much pain relief as you would get from a pill of oxycodone. So most people, when they practice mindfulness, are able to drop their pain by about one-third, but some people can reduce their pain by one-half or even more than that, and there are even some people who can completely alleviate their pain through mindfulness. When they practice mindfulness, their pain goes to a zero. We've heard reports like this time and time again from people going through this program, so I know that relief, and possibly even total recovery, from chronic pain is possible for you, just like it has been possible for the many people who have completed this program.

Now, to be clear, you can't expect the pain-relieving effects of mindfulness to last forever—they might wear off after a while. But using meditation to relieve pain is kind of like using medication. When you take pain medication and you get some relief, after a few hours the medication wears off, and then you need to take another dose. In the same way, after awhile when pain relief from mindfulness wears off, you have to take another dose of mindfulness to get more relief. But unlike medication, where often people develop tolerance and have to take higher and higher doses of the drug to get relief, with meditation, the more you practice it, the more relief you will get, and the longer that relief will last!

The practice of mindfulness is pretty simple. First, focus your attention on something. We usually start teaching mindfulness by encouraging people to focus their attention on their breathing, or a sensation in the body. But the object of mindfulness could be anything in front of you. It could be the sight of a beautiful sunset, or a flower in your garden. Choose something to focus on, and then just focus your attention only on that thing. If you are anything like me and many other mindfulness practitioners, you'll begin to notice in a few seconds that your mind starts to wander. Your mind might wander to random thoughts. It might wander to feeling like you want to fidget. It might wander to parts of your body that hurt. It might wander off into your memories about the past, or worries about the future. If the mind wanders, that's okay, that's what minds do. They wander. *When you notice that your mind wanders off, just notice where your mind has wandered off to, acknowledge and accept that thought, feeling, or distraction, and then bring your attention back to the point of focus.* We call that the "loop of mindfulness." [**Therapist note**: Show participants Handout S1.2 or draw the "loop of mindfulness" on a whiteboard.] That's it—that's the basic practice of mindfulness. Mindfulness is pretty simple—but that doesn't make it easy.

But remember, every time your mind wanders and you notice where it wanders off to, and you acknowledge and accept that thought, feeling, or distraction, and then you bring the focus of your mind back to the object of mindfulness (like your breath or sensations in the body), you've just strengthened your mind. That's why I said mindfulness is a form of mental training, like exercise for your brain. It's pretty similar to physical exercise. Have you ever lifted weights? If you want to make your bicep stronger, you curl a dumbbell, and every time you curl the dumbbell, your bicep gets stronger. [**Therapist note:** Demonstrate by doing an arm curl in the air.] Well, mindfulness is curling the dumbbell of the mind. So actually, each time the mind wanders gives you another opportunity to notice that it has wandered and then to refocus the mind. Each time that you do this, you are strengthening your attention, your self-awareness, and your self-control. You are strengthening the "muscles" of your prefrontal cortex to gain better control of your mind. A lot of people don't understand this—they think mindfulness is all about having a blank mind, and they get upset when the mind wanders. They think they are doing it wrong. But actually, mind wandering gives you a chance to practice mindfulness, to exercise the brain and get yourself back on track.

If you still don't really understand what I mean by mindfulness, that's okay. I promise you that it will start to make more sense once you begin practicing it. And, when you practice mindfulness, you will also start to experience its benefits. You will begin feeling a little more peaceful, a little more centered, and a little more in control. Mindfulness can reduce physical pain, emotional distress, and dependence on opioids. In fact, research shows that many people are able to use mindfulness to reduce their opioid use or come off their opioids entirely.

Mindfulness is a skill that can be learned through practice. Practice is really important, because the more that you practice a skill, the better you get at it—the more it becomes hardwired in your brain. It's just like learning any other skill, like riding a bike, playing sports, playing piano or guitar, or even learning how to read and write. When you were little, you didn't know how to do those things. You didn't even know how to tie your shoes! You had to learn them through practice. And at first it was hard to do these things. It might have felt awkward and unfamiliar. You had to concentrate, with a lot of effort. But over time, it became easier and easier. It's no different with mindfulness. The more you practice it, the better you will get at it. So now let's start with an exercise that will help you to understand what mindfulness is. I'm going to ask you to shift your attention around your body and become mindful of your body sensations.

Body Scan Practice[1]

Sitting comfortably . . . You can allow your eyes to close . . . or they can remain open and relaxed on a spot in front of you . . . You can begin by bringing your attention to the top of the head, to the scalp, just noticing the sensations there, whatever they are . . . And then letting them go . . . Moving the attention down to the forehead, just noticing the sensations there . . . whatever they are . . . And then letting them go . . . Moving the attention down to the muscles around the eyes, and the eyes themselves, just noticing the sensations there . . . whatever they are . . . And then letting them go . . . Moving attention to the inside of the head, to the center of the head, to the brain, just noticing those sensations there . . . whatever they are . . . And then letting them go . . . Moving the attention down to the jaw, the mouth, the lips, the teeth, the tongue, just noticing those sensations there . . . whatever they are . . . And then letting them go . . . Moving the attention down to the neck and the shoulders, just noticing the sensations there . . . whatever they are . . . And then letting them go . . . Moving the attention to the chest, to the heart, just noticing those sensations . . . whatever they are . . . And then letting them go . . . Moving the attention to the abdomen, to a point right behind your belly button, at the center of your being, just noticing the sensations there . . . And then letting them go . . .

Moving the attention to the low back, just noticing the sensations there . . . whatever they are . . . If you notice uncomfortable sensations, you can pay kind attention to them . . . And we have this word

---

[1] From *Mindfulness-Oriented Recovery Enhancement for Addiction, Stress, and Pain* by Eric L. Garland. Copyright © 2013 NASW Press. Adapted by permission of the National Association of Social Workers.

discomfort, *but what is it really? . . . Is it a heat? A tightness? A tingling? Are there thoughts or feelings associated with those sensations? And can you notice if the sensations have a center? Can you notice if they have edges? Perhaps the sensations are not solid . . . perhaps there are spaces inside the sensation, where the sensation is not . . . And if the sensation becomes too intense . . . You can notice where the sensation is not . . . Perhaps noticing the sensation of the air moving into the tip of your nostrils as you breathe . . . You can always return your attention back to the breath . . . As a way to recenter yourself . . . As a way to step back from sensation . . . And now imagine that you can breathe right into the intense sensations in the body . . . Sending the breath right into those sensations . . . to soften them . . . like water seeping down into soil . . . And then, letting those sensations go . . .*

Moving the attention to the hips, to the pelvis, just noticing sensations there . . . whatever they are . . . And then letting them go . . . Moving the attention to the thighs, just noticing the sensations there . . . whatever they are . . . And then letting them go . . . Moving the attention down to the knees, to the lower legs, to the calves, just noticing the sensations there . . . whatever they are . . . And then letting them go . . . Moving the attention to the feet, to the toes, just noticing the sensations there . . . And then letting them go . . . Then sweeping the attention as if it were a spotlight or a flashlight through the body . . . From the tips of the toes, to the top of the head . . . And from the top of the head, to the tips of the toes . . . From the front of the body to the back . . . And back to the front . . . From the inside to the outside . . . And from the outside to the inside . . . Then, expand the attention to encompass the whole body, becoming aware of the whole body, the whole body, the whole body . . . Then, perhaps becoming aware of space beyond the body, the space several inches above the top of your head . . . Then perhaps becoming aware of the space near the ceiling . . . In the corner of the room . . . Then perhaps becoming aware of the space above the ceiling, above the building . . . The space of the sky . . . And then perhaps becoming aware of the space beyond that . . . That's right . . . And now you can take one long moment to enjoy whatever positive feelings or thoughts have come up for you during this practice . . . or you can simply focus your attention on the breath or some other body sensation . . . That's right . . . Then, when a deeper part of your mind knows that each time that you practice this it will become easier and easier to go even more deeply into mindfulness, you may feel a little more comfortable, a little more centered, and a little more curious . . . when you complete this practice and bring your attention back to the room.

Process the Body Scan (Using PURER)

[Therapist note: PURER stands for phenomenology, utilization, reframing, education/expectancy, and reinforcement; see Chapter 5.]

What did you like best about that experience? Was there anything challenging about it? What did you notice in your body during this practice? If you found sensations of pain in your body, what did you notice about the pain as you focused your awareness on it? Did it stay the same? Did it grow stronger or weaker? Did it change in quality—for example, a burning became a warmth, a tightness became a tingling, and so on? Did you notice any thoughts or feelings about the sensations?

Relieving Pain by Zooming In

[Therapist note: If the session is running long, you can cover this material at the beginning of Session 2, right before you introduce the mindfulness of pain practice.]

The body scan might have made you feel a little better. But if you didn't notice any pain relief, don't worry—I haven't taught you how to use mindfulness to deal with pain yet. The main point here was to start to understand what mindfulness is about. The body scan is one way to learn to use mindfulness to become aware of and zoom in to sensations. Zooming in to sensations can actually help relieve pain. That seems counterintuitive, because we usually try to cope with pain by ignoring it or distracting ourselves from it, not focusing directly on the sensations. To understand how zooming in works, look at the image on Handout S1.3. [**Therapist note**: Give the group Handout S1.3.]

What do you see? Do you see a sad boy? Now if you were to zoom in with a magnifying glass, what would you see?

You would see that the image is made of pixels. When you are really zoomed in all the way, the "boy" is gone and instead all we find is little bits of shape and shadow. That's just like how we use zooming in to cope with pain. When we zoom in to the experience of pain, the "pain" is gone and instead all we find are sensations, like sensations of heat, or tightness, or tingling, as well as thoughts and feelings associated with those sensations. Our thoughts and feelings often get tied up in our sensations. Zooming in can help us to separate our thoughts and emotions about pain from the sensations themselves. It can help us to peel back the suffering that we lay on top of pain, which can actually turn down the volume of pain in the brain. And, when we separate out these sensations, thoughts, and feelings, coping with any one of them might be more manageable than coping with the overwhelming, anguishing experience of pain as a whole.

Zooming in also helps us to find the limits to our pain. Sometimes people feel like their pain is everywhere, like their whole body hurts. But when we zoom in, we might discover that the sensations are actually limited to only one part of the body. We start to notice the edges of the sensations—and that there are places in our body right next to the painful sensations that don't hurt at all. We might also notice that the painful sensations are not solid. If we zoom all the way in to them, almost as if our attention was like a microscope, we might notice that there are spaces inside the sensation where there is no sensation at all. It's kind of like what physicists have discovered about the atom: If you zoom in closely enough, you discover that the basic building block of matter is mostly made up of empty space.

Not only that, but zooming in helps us notice when sensations change over time. You might notice that the sensations start to fade away over time. Or maybe they first build to a peak, and then begin to fade away, like a wave rolling at sea. The sensations might also change in quality over time. A sensation of heat might change into a warmth, a tightness might change into a tingling, or a tingling might turn into a vibration, or an energy. Painful sensations change just like everything else in our bodies. Our bodies are in constant motion—things are constantly changing. Did you know that the brain changes every moment? The nerve cells in your brain are firing on and off constantly. That's why when we use electroencephalography (EEG) to measure electrical activity in the brain, the brain waves look like squiggly lines, wiggling up and down. Because the brain is always changing, and all pain is in the brain, then your pain can change, too. Using mindfulness to zoom in to pain can help us see that no sensation lasts forever. Realizing this fact can give us the strength to get through it. We are going to practice using mindfulness to zoom in as a way to relieve pain in future sessions.

Relieving Pain by Zooming Out

Another way to relieve pain is to use mindfulness to breathe in to the pain and then zoom out from it. To understand what I mean by that, we first need to learn the core skill of mindful breathing. Let's practice that right now.

Mindful Breathing Practice[2]

Sitting comfortably but regally, as if you are a king or queen, with your spine straight and belly relaxed, you can allow your eyes to close . . . or they can remain open and relaxed on a spot in front of you. You can begin to notice the sensation of the body resting in the chair . . . And you've been sitting in the chair for a while now . . . But now you can really begin to notice the sensation . . . of the legs and back making contact with the cushion of the chair . . . And we have this word contact, but what is it really? . . . A sensation of warmth? Or heaviness? Or tingling? Just noticing . . . whatever it is . . . just noticing the sensation . . . And when you are ready, you can begin to notice the sensation of the breath moving into the nostrils . . . And there's no need to breathe in any sort of special way . . . Just noticing the natural sensation of the breath . . . Noticing the temperature of that air . . . its warmth or coolness . . . That's right . . . And whenever the mind wanders to thoughts, emotions, images, or memories, that's okay, because that is what minds do—they wander . . . Just noticing where the mind has wandered off to, acknowledging that thought or feeling or distraction . . . And then letting it go . . . And gently but firmly returning the attention back to the breath . . . That's right . . . Each time that you notice that the mind has wandered, and you become aware of where the mind has wandered off to, and you acknowledge that thought and feeling . . . And then you return the focus of your attention back to the breath . . . You are learning to step back . . . to step back . . . to step back from your thoughts and feelings and into the clear, open space of mindfulness . . . You are strengthening your mindfulness . . . And soon you may begin to notice that thoughts and feelings come and go on their own, like clouds passing in a clear blue sky . . . Like clouds drifting, these thoughts come out of nowhere, gradually change shape, and then fade into the distance, all on their own . . . And there is no need to hold on to those thoughts or push them away . . . You can just let them go . . . And a part of the mind is like those thoughts passing like clouds . . . But there is a deeper part of the mind . . . that is more like . . . the space in which the clouds pass . . . the observing awareness . . . that is open . . . vast . . . perfect . . . and free . . . just watching, just observing . . . peacefully . . . And you can focus your attention on that part of your mind, or you can continue to focus your attention on your breath . . . That's right . . . And now, you can take a few long moments to focus on whatever positive experiences have come up for you during this practice . . . Appreciating and savoring those experiences now . . . or you can continue to focus on the breath . . . That's right . . . Then, when a deeper part of your mind knows that each time you practice this it will become easier and easier to go even more deeply into mindfulness, you may feel a little more comfortable, a little more centered, and a little more hopeful . . . when you complete this practice and return your attention to the room.

Process the Mindful Breathing Practice (Using PURER)

What did you like best about that experience? Was there anything challenging about it?

We talk more about mindfulness in the next session, and for the rest of this program—so it's fine if you don't fully get it yet. Just remember: It is totally okay if you noticed that your mind was wandering a lot. I really mean what I said: If you notice that the mind wanders, that's okay, because that's what minds do—they wander. Your mind doesn't have to be empty or blank in order to practice mindfulness. Mindfulness is all about noticing whatever is happening in the mind in this moment, and not holding on to it, or trying to push it away, but just watching it, like an observer or a witness. Once you become aware of a thought, feeling, or sensation in your body, you can just acknowledge and accept it, and then return your attention to your breath. This practice helps you to zoom out

---

[2]From *Mindfulness-Oriented Recovery Enhancement for Addiction, Stress, and Pain* by Eric L. Garland. Copyright © 2013 NASW Press. Adapted by permission of the National Association of Social Workers.

from your thoughts and feelings. If you found this exercise hard to do, don't worry about it. We will practice it over and over again, and eventually it will become easier. In doing this practice, you are strengthening your mindfulness, which will give you the strength you need to recover a good and meaningful life from pain.

[**Therapist note**: The section that follows lists the home practice assignment for the following week. Assign each bulleted point, and invite questions as needed to clarify the assignment.]

Home Practice

- Review Handouts S1.1–S1.5

- Daily mindful breathing or body scan practice

Try to practice about 15 minutes of mindfulness once a day with either mindful breathing or a body scan. If you don't have 15 minutes, then practice for three 5-minute sessions each day. If you miss a day, it's not a big deal. Just make sure to practice the next day. To learn the skill of mindfulness, I recommend that you find a quiet place to practice at a time when you won't be disturbed. Many people find that practicing at night before bed or right after they wake up are good times to practice. Once you get really good at mindfulness, you can do it anywhere: on a bus, on a plane, at work, or even in a stressful situation. Don't pressure yourself to achieve any kind of particular benefit, like feeling less stressed or experiencing pain relief. Just do the practice to get some experience with mindfulness. Whether or not you notice a benefit, you can know that your mind is growing stronger. Other benefits will come in time.

- STOP

The STOP practice is a brief technique to help strengthen your mindfulness. To practice STOP, you:

1. Stop before taking your opioid pain medication, or, if this is an issue for you, before you take another substance (drugs, alcohol) to get high.

2. Take a minute or two to practice mindful breathing to begin to quiet the mind and relax your body.

3. Observe your breath, thoughts, feelings, and sensations as they come and go for a minute or so. If you notice difficult thoughts, feelings, uncomfortable body sensations, or cravings, acknowledge them and return the focus of your attention back to your breath. Each time you do this, you are learning to step back, to practice "zooming out." You may feel a sense of distance from your medication or the drug, as if you were an observer or witness. And then . . .

4. Proceed with intention, deciding to take the medication (or substance), or not to take it. Whatever you decide is okay. You can decide to take your medication as usual. However, after practicing a couple of minutes of mindfulness, you might notice that your pain has subsided somewhat. So you might decide that you don't need to take as much opioid medication as you thought you did. Whatever you decide is right.

If you take medications for OUD like methadone or suboxone, you can use a variation of the STOP practice to increase your commitment to addiction recovery. In this version of the STOP practice, you: Stop before your medication. Take a few mindful breaths. Observe your breath, thoughts, feelings, and sensations; and then: Proceed by taking some time to remind yourself that you are taking a lifesaving medication. Bring to mind how being in recovery has made your life better, how it has helped you and the people you love. Think about how taking this medication is helping you to live a better, more functional, healthier, and happier life. Think about what you are grateful for.

This STOP practice is one of the most important in the MORE program. The purpose of this practice is to help you develop mindfulness about your opioid use. When you take an opioid or other drug, you are putting a powerful chemical in your body and brain. This is a serious action that deserves respect, attention, and awareness. Stopping before making this decision will give this action the respect and attention it deserves.

Common Pitfalls, Troubleshooting, and Closing Advice for the Therapist

This session, like all sessions, should close with the assignment of home practice. There are a few pitfalls to watch out for in this session. First, keep group participants on task during the discussion. Do not allow any one participant to give a lengthy disclosure, or you will run out of time. This session is very content heavy and if you allow for too much participant discussion or disclosure, you will run out of time to deliver some of the session content. The second pitfall is in relation to the expectation for pain relief in the body scan. The first time the body scan is introduced, the primary purpose is to help the patient gain insight into the nature of the pain experience as comprising sensations, thoughts, and emotions. We should not give the expectation for analgesia in this first mindfulness practice. If pain relief happens, that is wonderful, and you should provide reinforcement during the PURER process. But if there is no pain relief, make sure to communicate that the point of the practice is to increase mindfulness about the pain experience. Then, using PURER, build positive expectancy by communicating that even if the patient did not experience pain relief in this session, they are likely to achieve relief in future sessions with increased practice of mindfulness. Even without pain relief, they are strengthening their mindfulness. The final note to consider is that Session 1 is full of content. If you find yourself running out of time, just make sure to finish the body scan, process it with PURER, and assign the home practice. You can then skip the basic mindful breathing practice and instead give the psychoeducational material about "relieving pain by zooming in" and "relieving pain by zooming out" right before the first mindfulness of pain practice (which incorporates basic mindful breathing plus additional suggestions for zooming in and out from pain) in Session 2.

The experience most of us call "pain" is made up of several elements:

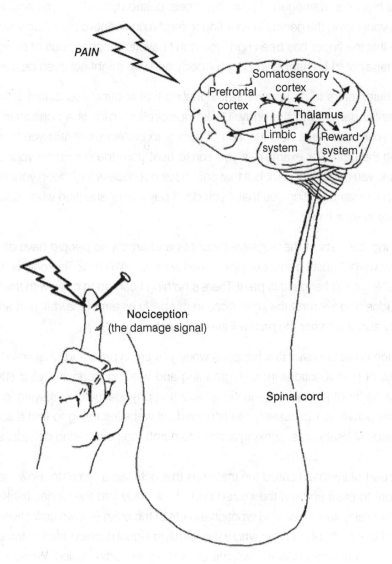

All pain is in the brain. The damage signal (nociception) is sent from the nerves in the body up the spinal cord into the brain, where the brain interprets this signal as the conscious experience of pain.

(cont.)

- **Nociception**, the "damage signal," sends information to the brain that the body has been damaged or is about to be damaged. That message is transmitted to the brain along nerves from the tissue that has been damaged. If your finger gets poked by a pin, or you accidentally touch a hot burner on your stove, the nerves in your finger send a nociceptive signal up your spinal cord to tell your brain that the finger has been hurt. You don't have to be conscious of nociception for this to occur; damage could be happening to your body and you might not even be aware of it.

- **Pain**, here, refers to an uncomfortable feeling that is often associated with some kind of actual or potential damage to the body. Unlike nociception, pain is a conscious experience: It occurs within your awareness. The function of pain is to protect us: It tells you to avoid the thing that is causing the pain. For example, if you sense heat from the burner on your stove, and pull your hand back, you might feel pain, but that pain does not necessarily mean your finger has been harmed. The pain may be telling you that if you don't pay closer attention when cooking, you may do real damage to your finger.

- **Suffering** consists of the negative thoughts and emotions people have about their pain. We suffer when we get upset about our pain, when we say, "Why me? This pain is ruining my life!" or when we think "I can't handle this pain! There's nothing I can do to cope with this!" We also suffer when we judge and interpret the sensations in our body as terrible, awful, and anguishing, and when we worry about whether the pain will ever get better.

- **Reaction** is the behavior that happens when you are in pain, and what you do to cope with pain. Examples of pain reactions include groaning and wincing, scanning your attention around your body looking for other painful sensations, avoiding physical activity, staying in bed, avoiding work and social activities, obsessively reading medical websites trying to find a solution to pain, seeking out medical treatments, drinking alcohol to numb the pain, taking opioids, and so on.

There's a part of the brain called the thalamus that acts like a "gate" to allow the damage signal (nociception) to pass up from the injured part of the body into the higher, thinking part of the brain, called the prefrontal cortex, and emotional parts of the brain (known collectively as the limbic system). It's in these parts of the brain where the damage signal is interpreted or translated as pain. You can think of the thalamus like the volume control on an audio device. When you change the focus of your attention, your prefrontal cortex can actually open up or close down the "gate" of the thalamus, which can increase or decrease the volume (or intensity) of the pain itself.

Mindfulness can help by decreasing suffering and negative pain reactions. But, mindfulness can also decrease the intensity of pain by reducing activity in the thalamus. In other words, mindfulness turns down the volume of the pain by closing the pain gate. Mindfulness reduces pain on average by about 30%. That's about as much pain relief as you would get from a pill of oxycodone. So most people, when they practice mindfulness, are able to drop their pain by about one-third, but some people can reduce their pain even more than that, and there are even some people who

(cont.)

can completely alleviate their pain through mindfulness. Now, to be clear, the pain-relieving effects of mindfulness don't necessarily last forever—you might find that they wear off after a while. But using mindfulness to relieve pain is kind of like using pain medication. When you take pain medication, and you get some pain relief, after a few hours, the medication wears off, and then you need to take another dose. In the same way, after a while when pain relief from mindfulness wears off, you have to take another dose of mindfulness to get more relief. But unlike medication, where people often develop tolerance and have to take higher and higher doses of the drug to get relief, with meditation, the more you practice it, the more relief you will get, and the longer that relief will last!

You can learn to reduce pain with mindfulness by (1) zooming in to pain and (2) zooming out from pain. Zooming in to sensations can actually help relieve pain. When we zoom in to the experience of pain, we may discover that the "pain" is gone and instead all we find are sensations, like sensations of heat, or tightness, or tingling, as well as thoughts and feelings associated with those sensations. Zooming in can help us to separate our thoughts and emotions about pain from the sensations themselves. It can help us to peel back the suffering that we lay on top of pain, which can actually turn down the volume of pain in the brain.

Zooming in also helps us to find the limits to our pain. Sometimes people feel like their pain is everywhere, like their whole body hurts. But when we zoom in, we might discover that the sensations are actually limited to only one part of the body. We start to notice the edges of the sensations—and that there are places in our body right next to the painful sensations that don't hurt at all. We might also notice that the painful sensations are not solid. If we zoom all the way in to them, almost as if our attention was like a microscope, we might notice that there are spaces inside the sensation where there is no sensation at all.

Not only that, but zooming in helps us notice when sensations change over time. You might notice that the sensations start to fade away over time. Or maybe they first build to a peak, and then begin to fade away, like a wave rolling at sea. The sensations might also change in quality over time. A sensation of heat might change into a warmth, a tightness might change into a tingling, or a tingling might turn into a vibration, or an energy. Painful sensations change just like everything else in our bodies. Using mindfulness to zoom in to pain can help us see that no sensation lasts forever. Realizing that can give us the strength to get through it. We will practice using mindfulness to zoom in as a way to relieve pain in future sessions.

Zooming out from pain helps us to cope by noticing the parts of our bodies and the parts of our lives that are not painful. When we notice the nonpainful (i.e., neutral) and pleasant parts of our bodies and lives, that makes the painful ones seem smaller by comparison.

The basic mindfulness-of-pain technique includes both zooming in and zooming out as ways of coping with pain.

Handout S1.2. The Loop of Mindfulness

Many people mistakenly believe that to be mindful means to be laser focused on the breath, without the mind wandering to any distracting thoughts, feelings, or perceptions (e.g., sounds). In reality, mindfulness involves *being aware of whatever is happening in the mind in the moment, and not trying to hold on to it or to push it away, but instead, just accepting and observing your experience, witnessing it unfold in the field of awareness.* So if thoughts, feelings, and distractions arise during the practice of mindfulness, that's okay, that's what minds do, they wander. You can just notice where the mind has wandered off to, acknowledge and accept that thought, and bring the focus of your attention back to the object of mindfulness (e.g., whatever you are focusing on, like the breath). That entire process, from focusing on the object of mindfulness, to noticing, acknowledging, and accepting mind wandering, and then to bringing your focus back to the object *is the practice of mindfulness!* Each time you go through this cycle (and you may go through many such cycles during a single mindfulness practice session), you are strengthening your mind's ability to become aware of itself. This capacity is known as *meta-awareness* (awareness of awareness). So it really doesn't matter how many times the mind wanders, because each time that it does, this gives you another opportunity to practice mindfulness. We call this cycle the "loop of mindfulness."

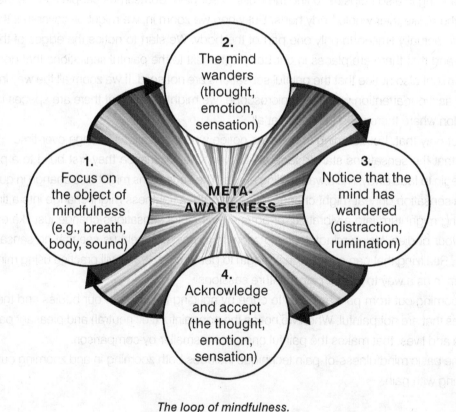

The loop of mindfulness.

Handout S1.3. Zooming in to Pain

To understand how mindfulness can help you to manage your pain, look at the images below.

What do you see in the image on the left? Do you see a sad boy?

Now if you were to zoom in with a magnifying glass, what would you see? Look at the image below on the right.

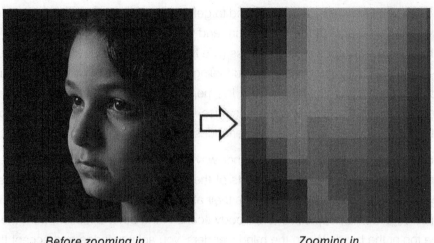

Before zooming in.　　　　　　　　　　　　　Zooming in.

      You would see that the image is made of pixels. When you are really zoomed in all the way, the "boy" is gone and instead all we find is little bits of shape and shadow. That's just like how we use zooming in to cope with pain. When we zoom in to the experience of pain, the "pain" is gone and instead all we find are sensations, like sensations of heat, or tightness, or tingling, as well as thoughts and feelings associated with those sensations. Our thoughts and feelings often get tied up in our sensations. Zooming in can help us to separate our thoughts and emotions about pain from the sensations themselves. And, when we separate out these sensations, thoughts, and feelings, coping with any one of them might be more manageable than coping with the overwhelming, anguishing experience of pain as a whole. We discover that a sensation is just a sensation, and sometimes, if we look deeply enough, a sensation might even be empty. Does the sensation have a center? Does it have edges? Are there spaces inside the sensation where the sensation is not? Use your mindfulness to see the true nature of sensation.

Handout S1.4. Mindfulness Practice

- **Mindful breathing.** Mindful breathing is a simple yet powerful practice. It involves focusing your attention on sensations of the breath (in the nostrils or in the abdomen). Pay attention to the temperature of the air, or to the rise and fall of your belly as you breathe. Some people prefer to focus on the sensation of air in their nostrils, whereas others like to focus on the movement of their diaphragm or abdomen. It doesn't really matter which point of focus you choose, and you don't need to change or control your breath. Just focus on the natural sensation of the breath. Soon you may notice that your mind begins to wander. Remember that if your mind wanders, that's what minds do, they wander! There's no need to get upset with yourself. When the mind wanders, you acknowledge and accept that distraction, and then return the focus of the attention back to the breath. After several loops of mindfulness (see Handout S1.2), you will find that you can "step back" or "zoom out" from your thoughts and feelings to observe them, witnessing them unfold in the field of awareness, moment by moment. In time, you may begin to start to perceive the space of awareness in which thoughts and feelings arise, and if so, rest your mind in that space. Then, appreciate and savor whatever positive experiences have come up during this practice.

- **Body scan.** The body scan is another way to practice mindfulness. It involves focusing your attention on sensations in various parts of the body and then accepting those sensations. During the body scan, one scans or sweeps their attention from the top of the head to the tips of the toes (although some people like to do body scans in the other direction, from the tips of the toes to the top of the head). When the mind wanders, you acknowledge and accept that distraction, and then return the focus of the attention back to the body part where you were noticing sensations. Once you have scanned your attention through the whole body, then become aware of the whole body, all at once. Finally, become aware of the space around the body and beyond the body. Rest your mind in that space. Then, appreciate and savor whatever positive experiences have come up during this practice.

- **Mindfulness of everyday activity.** Unlike mindful breathing or body scan, mindfulness of everyday activity does not require you to stop your normal activities to practice. On the contrary, it involves focusing your attention on your senses as you perform any one of your daily routine tasks (e.g., washing the dishes, taking a shower, sweeping the floor, preparing food for dinner, working in your garden, walking down the street). Pay attention to what you see, hear, touch, smell, and/ or taste as you perform this activity. Then, become aware of when your mind starts to wander into judgments, worries, or thoughts about the future or the past. When you notice that your mind is wandering away from the activity, acknowledge and accept the distraction, and then return the focus of the attention back into the activity. You may have to do multiple loops of mindfulness to stay focused in the present moment as you do this activity that you normally do on autopilot. Eventually you may find that you can stay focused and remain fully present for the entire activity. Appreciate and savor whatever positive experiences come up during this practice.

(cont.)

- **General mindfulness practice guidelines.** When you first start learning mindfulness, it can be helpful to find a quiet place to practice where you won't be disturbed. After you become more experienced, you can practice mindfulness in busy and noisy environments, or use mindfulness at times when you are under a lot of stress. You can practice mindfulness with your eyes closed or your eyes open. If you learn to practice mindfulness with your eyes open, you could be practicing in the middle of your everyday activity and no one will even notice! Also remember that the more you practice mindfulness, the better you will get at it—it's just like any other skill. If you don't have time to practice for a full 15-minute session, you can always have shorter practice sessions—they will still be beneficial. After you have been doing a 15-minute practice on a daily or near daily basis for a while, you may begin to notice that you can start adding in brief 3-minute practices in the middle of your day as a way to reawaken or refresh mindfulness whenever you need it to get a little extra relief from pain or stress, or when you want to become really focused or present.

Handout S1.5. STOP Practice

The STOP technique is a brief technique to help strengthen your mindfulness and inject some mindfulness into the middle of your day. To practice STOP, do the following:

1. <u>S</u>top before taking your opioid pain medication, your medications for OUD (e.g., methadone, suboxone), or, if this is an issue for you, before you take another drug to get high.

2. <u>T</u>ake a minute or two to practice mindful breathing to begin to quiet the mind and relax your body.

3. <u>O</u>bserve your breath, thoughts, feelings, and sensations as they come and go for a minute or so. If you notice difficult thoughts, feelings, uncomfortable body sensations, or cravings, acknowledge them, and return the focus of your attention back to your breath. And then . . .

4. <u>P</u>roceed with intention, deciding to take the medication (or drug), or not to take it. Whatever you decide is okay. You can decide to take your medication as usual. You might notice, however, that your pain has subsided somewhat. So you might decide that you don't need to take as much pain medication as you thought you did. Or, if you are taking medications for OUD, you might take a few moments to remind yourself that you are taking a lifesaving medication and remember your reasons for being in recovery.

Session 2

Mindfulness and Automatic Pilot

Agenda

Mindfulness-of-pain practice: 15 minutes

Process in-session mindfulness-of-pain practice (using PURER): 25 minutes

Process mindfulness home practice and STOP (using PURER): 15 minutes

Break: 10 minutes

Automatic habits in coping with chronic pain and stress: 20 minutes

Candy exercise: 15 minutes

Process candy exercise (using PURER): 10 minutes

Assignment for home practice: 10 minutes—discuss and assign for the following week:

- Mindfulness of everyday activity
- Daily mindfulness of pain or body scan
- STOP

Materials Needed

Chocolate or other candy for each group member

Paper towels to wipe hands clean

Handout S2.1. Mindfulness of Pain

Handout S2.2. Mindfulness of Everyday Activity

Session Introduction for the Therapist

This session, and every session thereafter, begins with the core mindfulness-of-pain practice. This practice builds upon the mindful breathing technique introduced in the last session by adding suggestions around the use of mindfulness to zoom in to and out of pain. The script for this mindfulness-of-pain practice does not vary from session to session. Instead, each session presents the same script, but the overall length of the practice increases from week to week as you increase the amount of silence in between each suggestion.

The session ends with the candy exercise. This practice aims to use mindfulness to increase awareness of automatic habits, and to use a safe metaphor to generate insight into the notion that one's opioid use can become an automatic habit, as well.

Session Script

Mindfulness of Pain[1]

Today we begin by learning the core practice of mindfulness to zoom in to and out of pain. This technique not only works to alleviate physical pain, it can also help to alleviate emotional pain when you are feeling stressed, angry, scared, or depressed. It involves focusing mindfulness on the sensations of your natural breath, and then becoming aware of any thoughts or feelings that come up for you. If your mind wanders to feelings of discomfort in the body, you can use mindfulness to first, briefly zoom in to the discomfort; second, imagine using mindfulness to breathe into the discomfort to soften it; and third, zoom out from the discomfort to watch it from the perspective of an observer or witness. You can use this practice anytime you are suffering from pain and want some relief. Let's try this now:

Mindfulness-of-Pain Practice

[**Therapist note:** This script is used at the beginning of each of the following sessions as the opening mindfulness practice. You may want to bookmark this page so that you can refer back to it easily.]

Sitting comfortably but regally, as if you are a king or queen sitting on your throne, with your spine straight, but not stiff, and your head held high, but your neck not straining . . . You can allow your eyes to close . . . or they can remain open and relaxed on a spot in front of you . . . You can begin to notice the sensation of the back and the legs making contact with the chair . . . And we have this word contact, but what is it really? . . . A sensation of warmth? Or heaviness? Or tingling? Just noticing that sensation . . . whatever it is . . . That's right . . . And when you are ready, you can begin to notice the sensation of the breath moving into the nostrils . . . And there's no need to breathe in any sort of special way . . . Just noticing the natural sensation of the breath . . . Noticing the temperature of that air . . . its warmth or coolness . . . That's right . . . And soon you may notice that the mind begins to wander . . . It may have already wandered . . . to thoughts, feelings, images, or memories . . . And if the mind wanders, that's okay, because that is what minds do—they wander . . . Just noticing where the mind has wandered off to . . . acknowledging . . . and accepting that thought or feeling . . . You might even say to yourself, "It's okay to have this experience right now, whatever it is" . . . And then, you can let it go . . . And then gently, but

[1] From *Mindfulness-Oriented Recovery Enhancement for Addiction, Stress, and Pain* by Eric L. Garland. Copyright © 2013 NASW Press. Adapted by permission of the National Association of Social Workers.

firmly, bring the attention back to the sensation of the breath moving into the nostrils . . . Back to the sensation of the breath moving deeper in the lungs . . . That's right . . .

And soon you may notice that the mind wanders again . . . to thoughts, feelings, or sensations . . . maybe even intense sensations that you normally label as discomfort . . . If you notice uncomfortable sensations, you can pay kind attention to them . . . And we have this word discomfort, but what is it really? Zooming in to those sensations now . . . Is there a heat? . . . A tightness? . . . A tingling? . . . Are there thoughts or feelings associated with those sensations? . . . Perhaps thoughts like "I don't like this," or "Why won't this go away?" . . . And can you notice if the sensations have a center? . . . Can you notice if they have edges? . . . Perhaps the sensations are not solid . . . perhaps there are spaces inside the sensation, where the sensation is not . . . And if the sensations ever become too intense . . . You can always notice where the uncomfortable sensations are not . . . You can always return your attention back to the breath . . . As a way to recenter yourself . . . As a way to zoom out from sensation . . . And now imagine that you can breathe right into those sensations . . . Imagining that you can send your breath right into those sensations, to soften them, like water seeping into soil . . . That's right . . . And then, return the focus of your attention back to the sensations . . . Can you notice how they are changing? . . . Perhaps the intensity is changing . . . Perhaps gradually getting weaker? . . . Perhaps becoming more intense, reaching a peak, and then gradually getting weaker, like a wave rolling at sea? . . . Perhaps the quality of the sensation is changing . . . Can that heat become a warmth? Can the tightness become a tingling? . . . Or an energy? . . . A vibration? . . . Or a spaciousness? . . . Perhaps the location is changing . . . You can notice if the sensations have a center . . . You can notice if they have edges . . . Perhaps the sensation is not solid . . . Perhaps there are spaces inside the sensation, where the sensation is not . . . And then you can let those sensations go, and gently return the focus of the attention back to the breath . . . Back to the sensation of the breath moving into the nostrils . . . Noticing the warmth or the coolness of that air . . . That's right . . .

Each time that you notice that the mind has wandered . . . And you become aware of where the mind has wandered off to . . . And you acknowledge and accept that thought or feeling or sensation . . . And then you return the focus of your attention back to the breath . . . You are learning to step back . . . to step back . . . to step back from thoughts and feelings and into the clear, open space of mindfulness . . . You are strengthening your mindfulness . . .

And soon you may begin to notice that thoughts and sensations come and go on their own, like clouds passing in a clear blue sky . . . Like clouds drifting, thoughts and sensations seem to come out of nowhere, change shape, and then fade into the distance, all on their own . . . And there is no need to hold on to those thoughts or to push them away . . . You can just let them go . . . And a part of the mind is like those thoughts and sensations passing like clouds . . . But there is a deeper part of the mind . . . that is more like . . . the space in which the clouds pass . . . the observing awareness . . . that is open . . . limitless . . . unbroken . . . and free . . . just watching, just observing . . . peacefully . . . And you can focus your attention on that part of the mind, or you can continue to focus your attention on the breath . . . That's right . . . And now, you can take a few long moments to focus on whatever positive experiences have come up for you during this practice . . . Appreciating and savoring those experiences now . . . or you can continue to focus on the breath . . . That's right . . . And when you know that each time you practice this, it will become easier and easier to go even more deeply into mindfulness . . . You may feel a little more comfortable, a little more centered, and a little more encouraged . . . when you complete this practice and return your attention to the room.

Process the Mindfulness-of-Pain Practice (Using PURER)

What did you like best about that experience? Was there anything challenging about it?

Process the Mindfulness Home Practice

How did you use mindfulness this week to help yourself with pain, opioid use (or addiction recovery)?

[**Therapist note:** The question about addiction recovery should only be asked if the group is comprised of people with OUD in recovery.]

Process the STOP Practice

When you were focused on your breathing, what did you notice about your attention for your medication? Did it keep getting pulled back to the sight of the medication? What did you notice in your body when your attention was focused on the medication? What thoughts did you notice? What did you do if you noticed your attention was captured by the medication?

If you don't have time to do the entire mindfulness-of-pain practice, but you are in pain and want to use mindfulness to help yourself, you could use the STOP practice to get in just a few moments of mindfulness before proceeding with your day. You might find that just a couple of minutes of mindfulness can do you some good. Many people in the MORE program report that the brief STOP practice can significantly reduce their pain in the moment.

Automatic Habits in Coping with Chronic Pain and Stress

When faced with physical pain or emotional distress, we do the best we can do to cope with the situation. Sometimes the way we cope is helpful. Sometimes the way we cope isn't so helpful—it might even make the pain or stress worse in the long run. When someone experiences pain or emotional distress day after day, they start to develop coping habits that often involve avoiding the things that make them feel worse. They may begin to avoid doing physical activity, being social, or going to work or school for fear that it will make things worse. They also might start using more opioid medication than prescribed, or start drinking alcohol or using other drugs to try to avoid feeling physical or emotional pain. Even though this kind of avoidance is completely understandable, it can make things worse. For example, when you avoid physical activity to prevent your pain from flaring up (something that many people with chronic pain do), over time you get out of shape, and this actually makes you more likely to become injured in the future.

People also develop mental coping habits. Some of these mental coping habits can be really helpful, like practicing mindfulness. But others aren't so helpful. Sometimes people try to ignore, suppress, or deny what is bothering them. Or, they tell themselves that their pain or stress is never going to get any better, and will probably get worse. Or, they start to blame themselves for their pain or stress, saying, "What's wrong with me that I have this condition?" Sometimes, people start to feel helpless and hopeless, telling themselves that they can't take action to make things better. Another kind of mental coping habit or reaction to chronic pain is to habitually scan the body for pain. For many people with chronic pain, the first thing they do in the morning when they wake up is to check their body to see whether their pain is still there or to try to figure out whether "today is going to be a bad pain day." It's actually pretty common for people with chronic pain to become hypervigilant, or on the lookout for pain. But when we use these sorts of mental coping habits, research shows that they can cause more emotional suffering. And emotional suffering can turn the volume of the pain up, making the pain even worse.

Do any of these ways of coping sound familiar to you? In what ways are they helpful, and in what ways are they not so helpful?

Early on, you might choose to use these unhelpful kinds of coping habits because you think they will be helpful. But over time, these kinds of coping become ingrained. You train yourself into them. People can be trained by giving them a reward when they do what you want. When you want a worker to do something on the job, you pay them a bonus. When you want kids to do their chores, you reward them with an allowance. It's not that different from when you want to train a dog. You want the dog to roll over, so each time it rolls over, you give it a doggie biscuit. Well, your reward was feeling less pain or less stress when you used your coping habit. For example, whenever you were hurting or feeling stressed out, and you took opioids to get some relief, you felt better, at least for a short time. So feeling better was the reward that reinforced your use of opioids. You trained yourself into the habit of opioid use, without even knowing it. Of course, you didn't do this on purpose. You did it unconsciously. You were operating on automatic pilot.

I'm sure you've experienced autopilot before. Have you ever gotten in your car and started driving, and then the next thing you know, you show up to where you were going without even remembering the drive? You were spaced out, lost in the clouds. You have no recollection of pressing the gas pedal or stepping on the brakes, changing lanes, going through intersections, stopping at stop signs, and passing people who were walking on the sidewalk. Of course you did all of those things and showed up to your destination safely, but you did them on automatic pilot. Because driving is such an ingrained habit, you can do it unconsciously, without even thinking about it.

When you do an action repeatedly, and that action is rewarded, it becomes a habit, and it starts to happen automatically, all on its own. Think about learning to tie your shoes. In the beginning you had to really think about how you could form one loop, and then another, and then tie them together. It was hard, and in the beginning, those loops often fell apart [**Therapist note:** Demonstrate with your own shoelaces.]. But over time, it got easier and easier, and eventually, became a full-on automatic habit, something you can do without even thinking about it. Just like that, you can use opioids, or other pain-coping habits, on automatic pilot. These automatic pain-coping habits are the reactions we were talking about in Session 1.

How do you relate this idea to your opioid use or other pain-coping habits?

Automatic habits have triggers. When you pull the trigger of a gun, the gun goes off. When an automatic habit is triggered, the habit goes off. If you are driving, and you see brake lights ahead, that's a trigger for you to step on your brakes. If a teacher asks you a question, and you raise your hand, that's a trigger for the teacher to call on you to answer. Triggers are often things that you see or hear or even smell, but they can also be feelings that activate a habit. For instance, if a person develops the habit of taking more opioids on days when they are stressed, the next time they feel stressed, that stressful feeling might trigger them to take an extra dose.

So you may have noticed when you did the STOP practice before taking your medication that your attention kept getting drawn back to the pill bottle or pills. Maybe you were trying to focus on your breathing, but then you noticed that it was hard to stop thinking about taking your medication. Many people experience that.

Did any of you notice this?

Maybe you have had the experience of doing some activity or being in a conversation and then having your pain flare up. Then you might notice that you are thinking about taking your medication instead of focusing on the activity or conversation you were having. You might try to refocus on the activity or conversation, but then find that your attention keeps getting pulled back to thoughts about the need to take your medication. It might become really hard to stop thinking about taking your next dose.

For someone who has taken opioids for a while, it is normal for your attention to be caught up by your pills. And when you find yourself focusing on your pills, it can make you want to take them. This is an example of the habit of opioid use being triggered.

Can you think of things that are triggers for your opioid use or other pain-coping habits?

In Session 1, we talked about mindfulness as a form of mental training, a way to strengthen the mind and become less reactive. Mindfulness is also a way to become aware of your triggers and gain control over your automatic habits. Think about it: When you practice mindfulness, you focus your attention on a point (like your breath). But then, after a few seconds, your mind starts to wander off automatically, and when it does, you catch it, and then bring your focus back. So in the same way, mindfulness can help you catch yourself when your attention is triggered and you start slipping into any automatic habit, and then help you bring your focus back to what you want to focus on. So if you are in the middle of a conversation or an activity and you find yourself in pain and fixated on thinking about when you can take your next dose of medication, you will become aware that your mind is wandering off, automatically. Then through practicing mindfulness you will have the ability to bring your focus back into the conversation or activity, to be more fully present with it so you can appreciate it more deeply.

Now we will practice an exercise that will help you to understand how mindfulness can increase awareness of automatic habits.

Candy Exercise

Begin by taking a few mindful breaths . . . Just noticing the sensation of the breath moving into the nostrils . . . Noticing the temperature of that air . . . Its warmth or coolness . . . That's right . . . Just noticing the natural sensation of the breath . . . And then, when the mind is a little more focused . . . a little more centered . . . a little more open . . . You can allow your eyes to open . . . And focus your attention on the piece of candy in your hand.

If the candy has a wrapper . . . You can slowly unwrap it . . . But don't eat it yet! . . . Once unwrapped, you can hold the candy up before your eyes . . . Paying close attention to it . . . Noticing it's color . . . it's texture . . . And as you turn the candy slowly to see all sides of it, perhaps noticing how it shines in the light . . . That's right . . .

Next, bring the candy to your nose and smell it . . . You can become aware of the precise moment when you notice the urge to eat the candy . . . But don't eat it yet! . . . And we have this word urge, but what is it really? . . . Zooming in to those sensations now? . . . Perhaps the mouth is filling up with saliva . . . Maybe you notice a feeling of hunger . . . or heat . . . or jitteriness . . . or tightness . . . or tingling . . . Perhaps your heart is beating faster . . . Maybe there are thoughts or feelings associated with those sensations, thoughts like "Why can't I just eat this thing?" or feelings of wanting or irritation . . . Observe that you can have an urge, but you don't have to give in to it . . . And if the mind wanders to thoughts, or feelings, or sensations, that's what minds do, they wander . . . You can just notice where the mind has wandered off to, acknowledging and accepting that thought or feeling, perhaps telling yourself in the space of your own mind, "It's okay to have this feeling right now," . . . whatever it is . . . And then you can let it go . . . And return the focus of your attention back to the sensation of the breath moving into the nostrils . . . Just noticing the temperature of that air . . . Its warmth or coolness . . . That's right . . .

Then, when you are ready, put the candy in your mouth, but don't chew it . . . You can become aware of the precise moment when the urge to chew the candy appears in your mind and body . . . But don't chew it yet . . . Notice the flavor of the candy in your mouth . . . Notice what it is like to experience an urge, but to not obey the urge . . . Then, when you are ready, start to chew, but chew slowly . . . Notice the flavor of the candy . . . Notice its texture . . . Becoming aware of the urge to swallow the candy, but don't swallow it yet . . . Just let the candy melt into your mouth, all on its own, naturally . . . Noticing what it's like to do that . . . Then, you can swallow if you wish, and notice the sensation of the candy traveling down your throat, into your belly . . .

Process the Candy Exercise (Using PURER)

What did you like best about that experience? Was there anything challenging about it? How might this experience relate to chronic pain and opioid use? Did you notice that your mouth and throat seemed to operate on autopilot?

Yes, it's amazing how many of our bodily functions and actions are controlled by autopilot. Once you start to bring mindfulness to your behavior, you will start to notice how much of what you do is being controlled automatically. In fact, some psychologists think that most of our actions as humans are happening unconsciously, automatically, all on our own, and that our conscious minds are not really in charge but instead are just "along for the ride."

What was it like to have an urge, but to not give into that urge?

Normally when we have an urge to do something, we just do that thing. No questions asked. If I'm thirsty, I drink. If I'm hungry, I eat. If I have an itch, I scratch. It's like the urge and the action are one thing. But really, that's not true. As a wise person once said, "Between stimulus and response there is a space. In that space is our power to choose our response. In our response lies our growth and our freedom" (Covey, 2010, p. vi). Practicing mindfulness can help you to become aware of when your urges are triggered. And then mindfulness can help you to be aware of the space between the urge and the action. Mindfulness can give you the freedom to choose to respond how you want to respond.

Did you notice when you were holding the candy that it was pretty hard to stop thinking about eating it?

Our thoughts and our attention can also be controlled on autopilot. But mindfulness can first help us to realize when something is triggering our attention and causing our minds to get stuck on that thing. Then, once we realize our minds have become stuck, we can use mindfulness to become unstuck by consciously shifting our attention back to the thing that we really want to be focused on. This is the skill of "zooming out" that we've been talking about and practicing. When you find your mind is getting stuck or fixated on something, refocusing your attention on the breath is a great way to break that cycle and zoom out.

Were you able to zoom out from the urge at all? When you did that, what happened to the urge?

We will keep working on that skill in the weeks to come, and in Session 5, I will teach you how to use mindfulness to overcome urges. For now, this exercise was really just intended to show you how your mind works when it goes on autopilot.

Mindfulness of Everyday Activity

You can increase your awareness of being on autopilot by practicing mindfulness of a daily activity. Think of something you do every day, some sort of routine action that you don't usually pay much attention to: maybe brushing your teeth or washing the dishes. It could even be something as simple as opening and closing your front door when you leave the house in the morning. See if you can focus your attention on your senses during this ordinary activity. Pay attention to what you see, hear, smell, and feel. Let's say you decide to try brushing your teeth mindfully in the morning. Notice the feeling of the bristles against your gums, the feeling of your fingers holding the brush, the smell of the toothpaste, the sound of the running water. When you notice that your mind starts to wander off to thoughts about what you are going to do later that day, what you are going to make for dinner, or what plans you have for the weekend, just acknowledge those thoughts, and then bring your attention back to noticing the scent of the toothpaste and the movement of your arm. See how long you can stay focused on the things you sense while brushing your teeth, before your mind wanders off. And don't get upset with yourself when your mind wanders; just notice it, and take it as an opportunity to strengthen your mindfulness. Then see if you can bring that same kind of mindful attention to this activity every day this week. Notice how your mindfulness of the activity changes over the course of the week.

Home Practice

- Daily mindfulness-of-pain or body scan practice
- Review Handout S2.1 Mindfulness of Pain
- Mindfulness of Everyday Activity (Handout S2.2)
- STOP (Handout S1.5)

Common Pitfalls, Troubleshooting, and Closing Advice for the Therapist

Note that this is the first time you present the candy exercise in MORE; the second time you will present a variation of this exercise is in Session 5. In Session 2, the candy exercise is presented as a means of increasing awareness of automaticity and potentially helping patients to gain insight into the habitual nature of their opioid use. Although you suggest that patients can become aware of craving in response to the candy, in Session 2 you are not providing any explicit instruction in using mindfulness to reduce craving. In contrast, Session 5 expands upon this technique by providing direct instruction in using mindfulness to regulate craving by zooming in, breathing in, and zooming out from craving combined with reappraisal (i.e., contemplating the consequences of indulging in the craving) and meta-awareness. Here, in Session 2, the candy exercise is a much simpler mindfulness technique—more appropriate for this early stage of the MORE program. Also note that this technique is sometimes confused with savoring. The intention of this technique is *not* to promote savoring of candy. Patients may begin to savor the candy, which is fine, but you should use PURER to reframe and redirect the conversation from talk of enjoying the candy to a discussion of awareness of automatic pilot and craving for the candy, and how this technique relates to opioid use. In our experience, at least one patient is likely to make the connection between their response to the candy and opioid use, which is often illuminating for others.

Handout S2.1. Mindfulness of Pain

You can use mindfulness to get relief from pain in three key ways. First, mindfulness can reduce the intensity of your pain, making it hurt less. Second, mindfulness can reduce the unpleasantness of your pain, making it bother you less. And third, mindfulness can give you the strength you need to tolerate the pain, helping you to get through it and remain resilient. Mindfulness can help relieve your pain in one or more of these ways.

When you are hurting, you can sit down and practice the full mindfulness-of-pain practice, which takes about 15–20 minutes to complete. In this practice, you begin with a few minutes of mindful breathing, and then focus your awareness on the uncomfortable sensations in the body. Remember, *discomfort* is just a word, but what is it really? Use your attention to "zoom in" to the experience of discomfort, and break it down in to sensations of heat, tightness, tingling, or other sensations. Notice if there are thoughts or feelings associated with those sensations. Then notice if the sensations have a center. Notice if they have edges. Notice if there are spaces inside the sensation where the sensation is not. Maybe the sensation is not solid. If the sensation becomes too intense, refocus your attention on your breathing as a way to "zoom out" from the sensation. Then imagine as if you could send the breath into the sensations, to soften them, like water seeping into soil. And then zoom back in to the sensations and notice how they are changing over time. Perhaps the intensity is changing (getting weaker, or first getting stronger and then getting weaker). Perhaps the quality of the sensations is changing. And notice if the sensations have a center. Notice if they have edges. Notice the spaces inside the sensation where there's no sensation at all. Eventually, notice how you can "step back" or "zoom out" from your sensations to observe them like a witness. Notice how sensations, like thoughts, come and go, all on their own, like clouds passing in a clear blue sky. Become aware of the space in which the clouds pass, the observing awareness, that is open, vast, perfect, and free, just watching and observing, peacefully. Rest your awareness on that part of your mind. Finally, take a few long moments to savor whatever positive feelings you have generated from this practice.

If you don't have a full 15–20 minutes, you could simply practice a few minutes of the basic mindful breathing practice to ease your pain. Remember, just like pain medication, the effects of mindfulness meditation don't last forever. When they wear off, you may need to "take another dose" by practicing a few more minutes of mindfulness. That's okay. You may find that with each time that you practice, the pain relief you get from mindfulness will get stronger and last longer.

Handout S2.2. Mindfulness of Everyday Activity

One of the best ways to increase awareness of autopilot is to practice mindfulness of a daily activity. To do this, pick something that you do every day, as a regular part of your day, some sort of routine action that you don't usually pay much attention to. Things like brushing your teeth, taking a shower, or doing the dishes are a good focus for this exercise. You could even choose something like opening and closing your front door when you leave to go to work. See how long you can stay focused on the activity before your mind wanders off. And don't get upset with yourself if your mind wanders; just be curious about it, and take it as an opportunity to strengthen your mindfulness. Do the same activity mindfully every day for the next week. Notice how your mindfulness of the activity changes from the beginning to the end of the week.

Here are the instructions for mindfulness of everyday activity:

1. Focus your attention on your senses during the activity. Pay attention to what you see, hear, smell, feel, and taste in the present moment during the activity.
2. When you notice that your mind starts to wander, just acknowledge and accept the distracting thought or feeling.
3. Then bring your attention back to what you are sensing about the activity (i.e., what you see, hear, smell, feel, and taste).
4. Repeat this cycle until you complete the activity.
5. Take a few long moments to savor the best parts of the experience. Rest your mind in whatever positive feelings have been generated from this practice.
6. Then, when you are ready, you can complete this practice.

Use the log below to record your mindfulness of everyday activity and what you noticed.

Date	Activity	What did you notice?
Example: 6-2-23	Washed dishes	The bubbles on the dishes, the movement of my arm, a feeling of peace

Session 3

Reappraising Adversity
as a Source of Growth

Agenda

Mindfulness-of-pain practice: 17 minutes

Process in-session mindfulness-of-pain practice (using PURER): 25 minutes

Process mindfulness home practice and STOP (using PURER): 15 minutes

Break: 10 minutes

Reappraisal story: 10 minutes

Mindful reappraisal of negative thoughts and pain: 10 minutes

Reappraisal practice: 18 minutes

Reappraising catastrophizing: 5 minutes

Assignment for home practice: 10 minutes—discuss and assign for the following week:
- Daily mindfulness of pain or body scan
- Mindfulness of everyday activity
- Daily reappraisal
- STOP

Materials Needed

Whiteboard or flip chart

Handout S3.1. Reappraisal Instructions

Handout S3.2. Reappraisal Worksheet

Handout S3.3. Example of a Reappraisal Worksheet

Session Introduction for the Therapist

The session opens with the mindfulness-of-pain practice first introduced in Session 2. Remember that the ideal moment to ask about the analgesic effects of mindfulness is when patients report experiencing some sort of a positive state in the mind or body (e.g., calm, peace, relaxation, joy, or bliss). Do this subtly by stating, "I'm just curious: When you experienced that positive feeling, what happened to your experience of pain in that moment?" Then, in this session, we build upon the foundational pillar of MORE, the practice of mindfulness, by introducing a new practice: reappraisal. Reappraisal, the second therapeutic pillar of MORE, is presented as a means of transforming negative thought patterns about stressors (including pain) and building resilience and meaning in the face of adversity. At the end of the session, you will discuss applying reappraisal to dealing with pain catastrophizing and addiction relapse. If you are not working with patients with OUD, you should omit the content around addiction relapse as it is not relevant to patients who have not progressed to that stage of opioid use.

Session Script

Mindfulness-of-Pain Practice

Use the practice on pages 100–101 in Session 2.

Process the Mindfulness of Pain Practice (Using PURER)

What did you like best about that experience? Was there anything challenging about it?

Process the Mindfulness Home Practice

How did you use mindfulness this week to help yourself with pain, opioid use (or addiction recovery)?

[Therapist note: The question about addiction recovery should only be asked if the group is comprised of people with OUD in recovery.]

Process the STOP Practice

When you were focused on your breathing, what did you notice about your attention for the medication/drug? Did it keep getting pulled back to the medication/drug? What did you notice in your body when your attention was focused on the medication/drug? What thoughts did you notice? What did you do when you noticed your attention was captured by the medication/drug? Did you notice that you could bring your attention back to your breath, and keep it there longer? Did you find that you were more disinterested in the medication/drug, like you just didn't care about it? Were you able to "step back" or practice "zooming out" during this experience? What was that like?

A Reappraisal Story

Today we will talk about another important practice in MORE. This practice is called reappraisal. Mindfulness teaches us how to observe and accept difficult thoughts and feelings. Reappraisal takes this process one step further by teaching us how to challenge and change upsetting thoughts to reduce painful emotions.

Changing the way we think about the difficult or painful parts of life can help us to cope with them more effectively. I'm going to tell you a story to illustrate this idea. This is the story of Grace. Grace has been suffering from chronic pain for the past 10 years. She has multiple herniated disks in her low back that hurt her a lot every day. She's not totally sure how she blew her disks out, but it probably was from repetitive strain from the physical labor she used to do at her job in the warehouse where she has worked ever since she got out of high school. Her pain and neuropathy became so severe that she finally got on disability, and stopped working altogether. One day her best friend convinced Grace to go back to community college to retrain for another line of work that wouldn't be so hard on her body—a good-paying desk job. She decided to study accounting, but accounting involves a lot of math, and some of those tests can be difficult. Grace hasn't taken a math class in many years, and so she feels really intimidated. She often wonders if she has what it takes to succeed in school. She often wonders if she is smart enough. She's afraid of flunking out and wasting all the money she has spent on classes. Then, one day she finds out she has a major math test the next week.

Based on what I just told you about Grace, do you think she believes she can pass this upcoming math test? If Grace believes she's going to fail the test, how would that thought affect her emotions? If she believes she is going to fail, how would that thought affect her actions? How likely is it that Grace would study a lot to prepare for the test?

But, there's a totally different way to think about this situation. Grace could be optimistic and believe that she can pass the test if she studies harder.

If Grace believes she can pass the test with enough hard work, how would that thought affect her emotions? If she believes she is going to pass with enough hard work, how would that thought affect her actions? How likely is it that Grace would study hard for the test?

As you might have guessed, Grace thought that she was going to bomb the test. When she started thinking about failure, she started getting stressed out and tense. And, feeling stressed and tense made the muscles in her back get very tight. Her worrying made her pain worse. Because her pain started to spike, Grace just wanted to lie on the couch and watch TV instead of studying.

What if, as an emotional reaction to the pain, Grace told herself, "There's no way I can study now. I'm hurting too much!" How would that thought affect her emotions? How would it affect her actions?

If Grace thought that way, she would start to feel hopeless and helpless. She might avoid studying, and her worries about the test might grow even stronger. She might even take an extra dose of opioids, just to take the edge off.

But there's another possibility here.

What if Grace told herself, "I know this test is going to be tough, and yeah, my back hurts, but I can still get some studying done. In the past I've been able to get stuff done in spite of my pain. The pain might make it harder to concentrate, but some studying is better than no studying. If I study, I'm going to feel better, and have a good shot of passing this test." How would that thought affect how she feels? If Grace thought that way, how would it affect her actions?

Fortunately, Grace chose to change her negative thoughts and think positively in this moment. When she told herself that she could take some action to prepare for the test, in spite of her pain, she started to feel more optimistic about passing. Not only that, she was so focused on the math that she didn't even notice the pain in her back and neck! When she finished studying, she felt more prepared, and so she relaxed, and the pain in her muscles decreased a little bit.

Mindful Reappraisal of Negative Thoughts and Pain

What's the moral of this story? In short, how we think about our life circumstances affects how we feel and the actions that we decide to take. This is a powerful idea, and a very old one, found in the sayings of ancient philosophers, such as Epictetus. Two thousand years ago he wrote, "We are disturbed not by events, but by the views which we take of them."

We can't control all of the events in our lives. And our emotions can be really hard to control. They often seem to come out of nowhere, like an afternoon thunderstorm that explodes with lightning and rain. But our thoughts are controllable. We can create any thought we want in an instant. Let me prove it to you.

If I tell you, "Think of a piece of pepperoni pizza," nod your head when you've done that. Now, "Think of some ice cream." Nod your head when you've done that. Now, "Think of a purple dancing bear, maybe with sunglasses."

[**Therapist note**: This is a practice—the therapist should pause and deliver these suggestions—and wait for a response.]

Consider our story. The way Grace thought about the upcoming test had a big impact on her emotions and actions. If she thought she couldn't study because of her pain, and then thought this meant she would bomb the test, Grace would feel really anxious and quite helpless and hopeless. Her back would hurt more, and she'd be really stressed. What might she do then? Sometimes, when people are stressed or experiencing other emotions like anger, sadness, or fear, they take more opioids than usual to help themselves feel better. That might work in the short run, but of course it can cause bigger problems, like opioid dependence.

Alternatively, if Grace thought she could be successful with enough studying, she would have felt calmer and more motivated to study, and probably could have gotten a better grade. Because she was less tense, she might have felt less of a need to take an extra dose of opioids. By studying for the test, Grace would probably also feel a sense of accomplishment and greater peace of mind knowing she had prepared.

When we are faced with a challenging situation, thinking negatively about the situation leads to stress. But interpreting life challenges more positively leads to feelings of calm and inner strength. Science shows that people who learn to positively reinterpret difficult life events are more resilient in the face of stress. And this happens even when people are confronted by serious disasters.

Do you remember in 2005 when Hurricane Katrina devastated New Orleans and much of Louisiana? When asked whether there were any silver linings to this terrible situation (Stanko et al., 2015), people who were coping well in spite of the catastrophic destruction said that Katrina had actually brought some good into the world by making people more compassionate. Strangers were helping strangers, out of kindness. They also thought that Katrina presented the opportunity to start a new life, an opportunity for better times ahead living in a different city. So seeing the silver lining in this way helped people to cope with the devastation.

Facing life's challenges can actually help us to grow. This way of thinking about challenges is useful for dealing with the many stresses that life throws at us. For example, if someone is laid off at work, they could see this as an opportunity to find a job they like more, or one that pays better. Or, if someone is diagnosed with high blood pressure, they could see this diagnosis as a way to jump-start healthy eating and exercise. Or, someone who experiences a drug overdose and survives could see this as an opportunity to turn their life around.

Can you think of any other examples?

Some really powerful, positive ways of thinking include:

- "Going through this challenge has made me stronger."
- "I've grown as a person as a result of facing this challenge."
- "I've become wiser and more compassionate by facing this challenge."
- "There's a silver lining here."

Changing the way we think about the difficult parts of our life is called reappraisal. Reappraisal reduces stress and increases our strength to cope with challenging life events. It's the key to resilience.

Mindfulness can help us to make reappraisals. Mindfulness calms down the mind, and makes the mind more open to new ways of seeing new perspectives on our life situation. Mindfulness can make our minds more flexible. Mindfulness is like WD-40 for your mind! It lubes up our thoughts when they are stuck, and helps us to reappraise difficult situations as learning experiences and opportunities for personal growth.

Reappraisal is a skill that can be learned through practice, just like any other skill. It can be broken down into a few steps (see Handout S3.1). When you are upset or stressed, you can follow those steps, as easy as A, B, C, D, and E:

A. What is the **a**ctivating stressor event? This is the event that led you to feeling stressed and upset. What happened during this event?

B. What unhelpful **b**eliefs or thoughts did you have about the activating event that led you to feel upset? Become mindful of any negative thoughts that you had in that moment when you were upset. Of those thoughts, which ones were the most upsetting to you?

C. What were the **c**onsequences of those negative thoughts? How did those thoughts make you feel? How did they affect your emotions, and the sensations in your body? How did those thoughts affect your actions? How did you react in that stressful situation?

Okay, great work, you are about halfway through this reappraisal process. The next step is to practice a minute or two of mindfulness, just enough to calm down your mind and your body, just enough to lubricate your thoughts, to get them unstuck. Remember, mindfulness is the WD-40 of the mind! Let's all practice a couple of minutes of mindfulness now:

You can just allow your eyes to close . . . or they can remain open and relaxed on a spot in front of you . . . And when you are ready, focusing your attention on the breath . . . On the sensation of the breath moving into the nostrils . . . Just noticing the temperature of that air, its warmth or coolness . . . That's right . . . Just noticing the natural sensation of the breath, in this moment . . . And if the mind begins to wander to thoughts, feelings, or memories, that's okay, because that is what minds do—they wander . . . Just acknowledging those thoughts and feelings, accepting them, and then letting them go . . . And then you can bring your attention back to the breath . . . That's right . . . Just noticing the temperature of that air, its warmth or coolness . . . Each time that you notice that the mind has wandered, and you become aware of where the mind has wandered off to, and you acknowledge and accept that thought and feeling . . . and then you return the focus of your attention back to the breath . . . you are learning to step back . . . to step back . . . to step back from your thoughts and feelings and in to the clear, open space of mindfulness . . . And soon you may begin to notice that the mind has become a little calmer, and little more spacious, a little more open . . . And then you can allow your eyes to open as your mind becomes more open to new ways of seeing this situation.

D. Now that your mind is more open to new perspectives, it is time to **d**ispute or challenge your negative thoughts, and come up with a reappraisal about the event. To do that, ask yourself the following questions:

- What's a more helpful way of thinking about this event?
- What is the proof that my negative thoughts about the event are true? What is the proof that they are not true?
- Is there an alternative explanation for what is happening here?
- What are some other ways that I could view this event?
- If I had a friend who was dealing with this same event, what would I want them to believe?
- If I had a spiritual advisor or teacher, what would they want me to believe?
- What are the positive aspects of the event?
- Is there a blessing in disguise here?
- Is there something to be learned from this event?
- How can facing this event make me stronger?
- How can going through this event bring a sense of meaning to my life?
- What can I do to make this situation better?

E. Last, what is the **e**ffect of your reappraisal? How would thinking this way affect how you feel? How would it affect what you do, what actions you take?

In the beginning when you start to learn reappraisal, you will go through the technique in a step-by-step fashion by filling out Handout S3.2. Even though we list the steps in order as A, B, C, D, and E, in reality a lot of times we start the process at C: We find ourselves experiencing emotional consequences, like stress, anger, worry, or sadness. Then we work backward and ask ourselves, "What just happened that led me to be upset?" That's A, the activating stressor event. Then we ask, "What was I thinking or believing about the activating stressor event that caused my upset feelings?" That's B. So now we know A, B, and C. Then we pause, and practice a minute or two of mindful breathing to calm down the body and allow the mind to become more open to new possibilities, new perspectives. And then we dive into D. We dispute and challenge the negative beliefs, and transform them into more helpful ways of seeing the situation—a positive reappraisal. Finally, we go to E and evaluate the effect of the reappraisal.

Eventually, when you get really good at this practice, you will be able to do the steps rapidly in your mind. You won't even need to write anything down. You may find that you can use mindfulness to rapidly catch yourself when you are starting to fall into a downward spiral of negative thinking, and stop it in its tracks. Then you can challenge and change those negative beliefs into a positive reappraisal, even before you get very stressed or upset. In time you'll be able to use reappraisal to prevent yourself from becoming too reactive. But this takes practice, so let's practice the skill of reappraisal now.

Reappraisal Practice

[**Therapist note:** Demonstrate the process of reappraisal by asking the group if anyone can volunteer and give an example from the past week when they felt "upset, angry, sad, worried, or stressed. Not something too stressful, but something about a 3 on a scale of 0–10, with 0 being not stressful at all, and 10 being the most stressful thing imaginable." Using a whiteboard (or Handout S3.2), draw the five rows (A, B, C, D, and E) from the Reappraisal Worksheet (Handout S3.2) and fill them out with details from the example given in group—beginning with row C. Once rows A, B, and C are complete, the clinician should guide the group in practicing 2–3 minutes of mindful breathing before continuing on to rows D and E. The clinician should then ask the volunteer questions listed under D to facilitate disputation of the negative thoughts and the formation of a new positive reappraisal. If the volunteer has difficulty generating disputations, the clinician should turn to the group for support and advice in step D.]

Reappraising Catastrophizing

Reappraisal isn't just useful for dealing with stress. It can also help us to deal with pain. When someone experiences a pain flare-up, they often believe their condition is getting worse. Then they might start to worry that the pain is never going to go away. They might think there is nothing they can do to make the pain better, and they start feeling hopeless. Thinking this way leads to feelings of sadness and worry, negative emotions that can actually turn up the volume of the pain by changing the way pain is processed in the brain. This kind of thinking is called catastrophizing. Research shows that catastrophizing increases pain and disability. And when people catastrophize, they are more likely to take higher and higher doses of opioids just to feel okay.

But, just like in our story of Grace, it's possible to think more positively about pain. Instead of catastrophizing, a person could think, "I'm having a pain flare-up, but I've had them before, and they've always settled down over time. This one will settle down too. Until it does, I can do things to manage the pain and make myself feel better."

If someone thought that way, how would it affect how they feel? How would it affect their actions?

So reappraisal can be useful for overcoming pain catastrophizing. If you experience a pain flare-up and start to feel upset or worried about the pain, you can use the *ABCDE* approach that we just talked about. Become aware of the negative beliefs and thoughts you are having about pain. Practice a few minutes of mindfulness to calm down and open the mind to new perspectives. Then ask yourself the following questions:

- What's a more helpful way to think about this pain flare-up?
- What's the proof that this pain flare-up is never going to get better? What's the proof that it might get better?
- What are some things that I can do to make it better?
- If my friend was experiencing a pain flare-up like this, what would I want them to believe?
- If I had a spiritual advisor or teacher, what would they want me to think about this pain flare-up?
- Has facing pain taught me something, made me stronger, or brought some sort of meaning to my life?

That last question is a tough one. But it's worth asking. Sometimes people realize that having chronic pain has made them more appreciative, more compassionate, more resilient, and more grateful.

Once you've reappraised in this way, you can shift your attention to something more helpful or positive, like doing one of your favorite hobbies, getting some light exercise, taking care of some things around the house, or spending time with someone who really cares about you. If your mind starts to wander back to catastrophizing, take a few mindful breaths, and gently remind yourself of your reappraisals.

[Therapist note: This next section is relevant only if there are people in recovery from OUD in your group. If your group has no one in recovery, omit this material.]

Catastrophizing also happens during addiction recovery. When people try to change an unhealthy habit like addiction to opioids, or drinking too much, smoking, overeating, and so on, they don't just change all at once. In fact, often, people relapse back to the old habit several times before breaking the habit. Change doesn't just happen in a straight line of progress. Sometimes you take two steps forward, one step back, then one step forward, two steps back, and then two steps forward, and one step back. Eventually, you get one step ahead, and that's a step closer to achieving your goal!

It's important to recognize that relapses are part of the recovery process. Sometimes, when someone in recovery has been off drugs for a while, and then because of stress or peer pressure, or being triggered, they get high. When that happens, sometimes people think things like "Damn, I just totally screwed up. I just blew my recovery. I'm a loser. Now that I just ruined everything, I might as well go back into my addiction." This kind of thinking is another form of catastrophizing that can lead to self-destructive behavior. But, you can use reappraisal in this situation, too. You can realize that just because you fell off the wagon, doesn't mean that you have to stay down in the dirt. Just because you used drugs once, doesn't mean you have to use them again. Instead, you can pick yourself back up, dust yourself off, and get back on the wagon, to ride and enjoy another day.

If there is time, assess patient motivation by asking the following:

How are you feeling about the program (and skills) so far? How is this helping? What do you like the best? How are you feeling about continuing? What can I do to help you get more out of this course and achieve your goals?

Home Practice

- Daily mindfulness-of-pain or body scan practice
- Mindfulness of one daily activity
- Daily reappraisal practice (with Handout S3.2)
- STOP (Handout S1.5)
- Bring an item to the next session for the savoring exercise (e.g., flower, art, photograph, object with positive associations)

Common Pitfalls, Troubleshooting, and Closing Advice for the Therapist

Remember to have the volunteer for the reappraisal exercise choose a stressful event that is about a 3 on a scale of 0–10. You do not want the patient to bring up extreme stressors like sexual assault, the death of a loved one, homelessness, and so on that you cannot easily help them to reappraise within the 18 minutes allotted to this exercise during the session. The ideal situation for reappraisal is one in which the patient is likely catastrophizing or thinking irrationally, leading to negative emotions that may be out of proportion with the actual stressor. Of course, reappraisal can be used to address more severe stressors, but given the context of the group and limited amount of time you have to complete this technique, it's best to select a more manageable example that can be fully addressed in the time available.

Handout S3.1. Reappraisal Instructions

Reappraisal is an effective way to deal with negative thoughts and emotional distress. Reappraisal involves challenging and changing negative thought patterns to decrease emotional pain and suffering. When you make a reappraisal, you think about whatever situation is upsetting you in a different way, in a way that makes you feel more at peace, more empowered, or even more grateful. To reappraise, it's as simple as *ABCDE*!

Here are the basic reappraisal instructions. When you are upset or stressed, follow these steps:

A. What is the **a**ctivating stressor event? This is the event that led you to feel stressed and upset. What happened in this event?

B. What unhelpful **b**eliefs or thoughts did you have about the activating event that led you to feel upset? Become mindful of any negative thoughts that you had in that moment when you were upset. Of those thoughts, which ones were the most upsetting to you?

C. What were the **c**onsequences of those negative thoughts? How did those thoughts make you feel? How did they affect your emotions, and the feelings in your body? How did those thoughts affect your actions? How did you react in that stressful situation?

Now, practice a minute or two of mindfulness, just enough to calm down your mind and your body, just enough to lubricate your thoughts, to get them unstuck. Remember, mindfulness is the WD-40 of the mind! Let's all practice a couple of minutes of mindfulness now:

Close your eyes and focus on the sensations of the breath in your nostrils or in your abdomen. When the mind wanders, that's okay. Just notice, acknowledge, and accept that thought or feeling. Then let it go and return the focus of your attention back to the breath. And when the mind becomes open to new ways of seeing this situation, you can open your eyes.

D. Now that your mind is more open to new perspectives, it is time to **d**ispute or challenge your unhelpful thoughts, and come up with a reappraisal about the event. To do that, ask yourself the following questions:

What's a more helpful way of thinking about this event?
What is the proof that my negative thoughts about the event are true? What is the proof that they are not true?
Is there an alternative explanation for what is happening here?
What are some other ways that I could view this event?

(cont.)

If I had a friend who was dealing with this same event, what would I want them to believe?

If I had a spiritual advisor or teacher, what would they want me to believe?

What are the positive aspects of the event?

Is there a blessing in disguise here?

Is there something to be learned from this event?

How can facing this event make me stronger?

How can going through this event bring a sense of meaning to my life?

What can I do to make this situation better?

Reappraisals are your more helpful thoughts and positive ways of viewing the event.

E. Last, what is the **e**ffect of your reappraisal? How would thinking this way affect how you feel? How would it affect what you do and what actions you take?

Use Handout S3.2 to walk yourself through this practice in a structured way.

Handout S3.2. Reappraisal Worksheet

Before filling out this blank copy, see Handout S3.3, Example of a Reappraisal Worksheet. Then make as many blank copies as you need and practice reappraisal regularly!

Date: _____

A. **Activating stressor event:**

_____

_____

B. **Unhelpful beliefs or thoughts about the event:**

_____

_____

_____

C. **Consequences of the beliefs or thoughts:**

_____

_____

_____

MINDFUL BREATHING

D. **Dispute, challenge, and reappraise the unhelpful thought:**

_____

_____

_____

_____

_____

E. **Effect of the reappraisal:**

_____

_____

Here's an example of how to use the Reappraisal Worksheet.

Date: __4/28/23__

A. **Activating stressor event:**

   __My back started hurting more after my physical therapy appointment.__

B. **Unhelpful beliefs or thoughts about the event:**

   __"I must have hurt myself. Now my back is screwed." "I can't handle this."__

   __"There's nothing I can do to make this better."__

C. **Consequences of the beliefs or thoughts:**

   __Anger. Worry. Stop doing my PT [physical therapy] exercises.__

   __Took an extra dose of oxycontin.__

MINDFUL BREATHING

D. **Dispute, challenge, and reappraise the unhelpful thought:**

   __"My PT [physical therapist] tells me that it's normal to feel sore after doing the exercises.__

   __It means I'm restoring my function." "I've had many back flare-ups before and I've__

   __gotten through them. I can get through this one." "Mindfulness helps reduce my pain.__

   __It's worked before so it will work again."__

E. **Effect of the reappraisal:**

   __Less angry. Not sad. Calm. More motivated to do PT. Took a slow and gentle walk__

   __around my neighborhood.__

Session 4

Savoring Healthy Pleasure, Joy, and Meaning in Life

Agenda

Mindfulness of pain practice: 20 minutes

Process in-session mindfulness-of-pain practice (using PURER): 10 minutes

Process mindfulness home practice and STOP (using PURER): 10 minutes

Process reappraisal home practice (using PURER): 20 minutes

Break: 10 minutes

Smell the roses or feel the thorns: 10 minutes

Savoring the good: 10 minutes

Savoring practice: 10 minutes

Process savoring practice (using PURER): 10 minutes

Assignment: 10 minutes—discuss and assign for the following week:
- Daily mindfulness of pain or body scan
- Daily reappraisal
- Daily savoring
- STOP

Materials Needed

Objects for mindful savoring exercise (e.g., flowers, photographs, art, polished stones, fruit)

Handout S4.1. Zooming Out

Handout S4.2. Savoring

Session Introduction for the Therapist

In this session, we introduce the third therapeutic pillar of MORE: savoring. Savoring is one of the most vitally important and therapeutically potent components of MORE. Savoring is presented as a means of noticing pleasant events, boosting positive emotions, amplifying natural healthy pleasure, finding meaning in life, and eliciting experiences of self-transcendence: the sense of interconnectedness between the self and the world. To seed these concepts, focus your PURER processing of the introductory mindfulness of pain practice on helping patients to identify and appreciate positive emotions and pleasant body sensations arising during mindfulness.

Session Script

Mindfulness-of-Pain Practice

Use the practice on pages 100–101 in Session 2.

Process the In-Session Mindfulness-of-Pain Practice (Using PURER)

What did you like best about that experience? Was there anything challenging about it?

Process the Mindfulness Home Practice

How did you use mindfulness this week to help yourself with pain, opioid use (or addiction recovery)?

[**Therapist note:** The question about addiction recovery should only be asked if the group is comprised of people with OUD in recovery.]

Process the STOP Practice

When you were focused on your breathing, what did you notice about your attention for the medication/drug? Did it keep getting pulled back to the medication/drug? What did you notice in your body when your attention was focused on the medication/drug? What thoughts did you notice? What did you do when you noticed your attention was captured by the medication/drug? Did you notice that you could bring your attention back to your breath, and keep it there longer? Did you find that you were more disinterested in the medication/drug, like you didn't care as much about it? Were you able to "step back" or practice "zooming out" during this experience? What was that like?

Process the Reappraisal Home Practice

Can you tell me about your practice of reappraisal this week? Let's walk through another example. [**Therapist note:** Demonstrate the process of reappraisal by asking the group if anyone can volunteer and give an example from the past week when they felt "upset, angry, sad, worried, or stressed. Not something too stressful, but something about a 3 on a scale of 0–10, with 0 being not stressful at all, and 10 being the most stressful thing imaginable." Using a whiteboard (or Handout S3.2), draw the five rows (*ABCDE*) from the Reappraisal Worksheet and fill them out with details from the example given in group. Once rows *A*, *B*, and *C* are complete, the clinician should guide the group in practicing 2–3 minutes of mindful breathing before continuing on to rows *D* and *E*. The clinician should then ask the volunteer questions listed under *D* to facilitate disputation of the negative thoughts and the formation of a new positive reappraisal. If the volunteer has difficulty generating disputations, the clinician should turn to the group for support and advice in step *D*.]

Smell the Roses or Feel the Thorns?

As you know, when someone is dealing with chronic pain or is experiencing problems with opioids, they often feel pretty bad. And when you feel bad, it's natural to start paying more and more attention to the bad feelings. The problem is that the more you are on the lookout for bad feelings, the worse you feel. It might start to seem like all you can feel is physical and emotional pain. You might start to think "Life sucks! I always feel like crap!"

But if we start to pay mindful attention to life, we can begin to notice that even during the worst pain flare-ups, terrible pain or negative emotions aren't there every single second of the day. It might feel that way, but if we pay careful attention and are mindful to the moment-by-moment changes in life, we can discover that there are always moments, no matter how brief, when we are not in awful pain and agony. In those moments, we might be so focused on what we are doing that we might not even be noticing our pain at all. In that moment, our pain is temporarily gone! It's a moment of relief.

When have you experienced this before?

We often miss these little moments of feeling good because the painful parts of life automatically capture our attention. That's part of the autopilot we discussed in Session 2. Have you heard the phrase "stop and smell the roses"? We often don't do that, because we are feeling life's thorns instead. We tend to miss the roses and instead focus on the thorns because of the way our brains are wired by evolution. Our cavemen ancestors needed to be constantly on the lookout for danger to survive in a world full of prehistoric monsters like cave bears and saber-toothed tigers. But in the world we live in today, there are no giant monsters to fight. Staying hyperfocused on danger can stress us out and turn the volume of our pain way up.

So the way our brains evolved makes it more likely that we focus on the negative parts of life, especially when we are in pain or struggling with addiction. Chronic pain and long-term opioid use can actually make the brain more sensitive to stress and negativity, and less sensitive to natural healthy pleasure. I don't know if you can relate to this. Maybe this has happened to you before, or maybe it hasn't. But, when these brain changes get bad enough it can put the person in a hole, and they might start to feel empty inside. And so sometimes people start to take higher and higher doses of opioids just to feel okay. But then taking higher doses of opioids makes the brain even more sensitive to negative experiences, and even less sensitive to natural healthy pleasure, joy, and meaning in life. This pattern becomes a vicious cycle—a downward spiral that leads to increasing dependence on opioids. Eventually, we may start to feel like pain and addiction have robbed us of everything good in our lives. But we aren't helpless victims of our biology. We have a choice about where we focus our attention. From a philosophical perspective, why should we treat the negative parts of our life as more deserving of our attention than the positive parts of life, than the things we really care about or find meaningful?

As Viktor Frankl, a Holocaust survivor who lived through the Nazi concentration camps, once said, "Everything can be taken from a man but one thing: the last of the human freedoms—to choose one's attitude in any given set of circumstances" (1946/1959, p. 86). Though we are wired to be on the lookout for danger, we can use mindfulness to choose to focus on what we want to focus on, to have an attitude of appreciation for the good in our lives, in spite of the pain. Mindfulness can help us to notice and savor the moments of goodness around us.

Although we may not notice them, there are little moments that happen each day when things aren't completely awful. In those moments, you might be really focused on and fascinated by something pleasant that is happening—you might be watching a movie that you love, enjoying your favorite song, or maybe even listening to a bird singing outside your window. Sometimes, in those moments, you might not notice your physical or emotional pain. You are just so absorbed in the moment that you forget all about it. For that moment, the pain isn't a big deal, or maybe, for a split second, the pain isn't even there. If you really start paying mindful attention, you will discover that these little moments happen all the time. Even on the worst of days, there are good things going on in your life. However, we often don't notice or appreciate them, because we are operating out of automatic pilot.

I'll give you an example that many people can relate to. Have you ever had the experience of eating one of your favorite foods, but then you get so distracted by the conversation happening next to you, or by what's on your mind, that the next thing you know, you look down and realize you finished the food without even remembering what it tasted like? Maybe you enjoyed the first bite, but then your mind wandered off, and meanwhile, you kept on eating mindlessly. So now the food's all gone, and you didn't even get a chance to enjoy it!

As you continue on your journey of recovery from pain or addiction, it's really important to use mindfulness to notice and appreciate the moments in life when you are not feeling quite as bad, or maybe even feeling pretty good. You can use mindfulness to start to catch even the smallest glimpses of feeling good. Like on a cloudy day when the sun starts peeking through the clouds, and just for a moment, you enjoy the warmth of the sunshine on your face. When you start to notice those little moments of feeling good, you can become aware of what you are thinking and what you are doing in those moments of goodness. You might even want to write down a list of the positive things that you experience, think, and do each day. If you write down three things each day on your list, that's 21 positive moments a week, 90 in a month, and over 1,000 in a year! Then you can refer back to that list the next time you are feeling down, to get a bit of sunshine on a cloudy day.

But mindfulness isn't only useful for noticing the moments when you feel good. You can also use mindfulness to deeply focus on the pleasant experiences in your life, and to extract every little bit of pleasure that you can out of the moment.

Savoring the Good

You have been learning how to use mindfulness to bring close attention to your breath and to sensations in your body. You can use it to zoom in to any discomfort you feel. But you can also use mindfulness to zoom out—to shift your attention away from pain and unpleasant feelings, and toward the good things in your life. We call this practice *savoring*. You can use it to focus your attention on a pleasant object or event, and then to appreciate and absorb all of the positive feelings that experience has to offer. In this practice, you become mindful of your senses—what you see, hear, feel, smell, and taste—instead of getting caught up in your thoughts. If you really think about it, a lot of the time we aren't really sensing the world around us—instead, we are lost in daydreams. Sometimes we get so caught up in our thoughts, feelings, and memories that we lose contact with the world around us. Maybe you've had the experience of losing your keys and frantically searching your home for them, only to discover they were right there in your pocket or purse. These kind of things can happen easily when you have a lot on your mind. When you are lost in thoughts about pain or the stressful things in your life, you start to overlook the little moments of beauty all around you. Nonetheless, that beauty is there, just waiting to be noticed.

Have you ever savored the variety of flavors and textures in a nice meal? Maybe you were at a fancy restaurant, or someone made you your favorite food for your birthday, and you have this delicious morsel in front of you. You want to really enjoy it. So instead of wolfing it down, you admire how delicious the food looks, and take a few moments to take in its aroma. Then you eat it slowly, taking one bite at a time, tasting every little bit of it, rolling it around on your tongue, noticing how your body tingles with delight as you relish every bite. It turns out you can do that with other things, besides food. You can learn to savor all sorts of everyday pleasures and positive life experiences.

When we savor, we can taste the goodness in our life. There is so much pleasure and satisfaction in life to be found when we are not hyperfocused on physical and emotional pain. And, savoring helps us to step back from pain and negative thoughts and emotions—it can help us to disrupt automatic pilot and really live in the now.

Research also shows that when people feel happy, their physical and emotional pain hurts less. Focusing on feeling good can actually reduce pain-related activation in the brain. Research shows that when we feel happy, the reward center of the brain (the striatum) becomes activated, and the brain releases endorphins—your body's own pleasure chemical and a kind of natural opioid—a natural pain reliever. So when we savor positive feelings in the mind and the body, this can cause the brain to release more endorphins, which can reduce your pain!

Not only that, savoring is a way to make yourself feel better, naturally. In fact, several research studies have shown that training in savoring can actually make your brain and body become more sensitive to natural healthy pleasure. And the more sensitive the brain and body become to natural healthy pleasure, the less of a need people feel for opioids! Savoring can actually reduce the need you feel for opioids. Neuroscience shows that savoring increases activity in the brain's reward and pleasure circuits, in the same parts of the brain that are activated by drugs like opioids. If you can use savoring to stimulate your brain's pleasure centers, your brain can produce its own natural, internal opioids, and then maybe you won't need to take as much external opioid medication to experience the relief and comfort that you want to feel!

Savoring can also help us to cope with the painful parts of our life. When we are experiencing pain or something stressful, that painful or stressful event becomes the center of our focus, and we ignore the parts of our life that are positive or maybe not so bad. We become laser focused on the painful or stressful thing—it's a kind of tunnel vision. That painful or stressful thing becomes the sole focus of our awareness—it's all we see. [**Therapist note**: Give the group Handout S4.1 to illustrate this point.]

But we can learn to use mindfulness to zoom out from this tunnel vision, and expand the field of our awareness to encompass not only the painful or distressing parts of life but also the many neural and positive events and experiences that occur on a daily basis. Mindfulness gets us out of the tunnel by expanding our vision. And then we can begin to practice savoring by noticing and appreciating the positive aspects of our life. And when we do that, the painful parts of our life become smaller by comparison. The negative things can still be there, but they are no longer a central focus. They can start to fade into the background. [**Therapist note**: Refer to Handout S4.1 to illustrate this point.]

You can learn to practice savoring, just like any other skill. Here's how you do it. Choose an object to savor, something that you find beautiful, or life affirming, or meaningful. It could be something that looks beautiful, like a flower, a beautiful landscape, a sunset, or a mountain. It could be something that sounds good, like the sound of the wind through the trees or the song of a bird, or maybe even your favorite music. It could be something that feels pleasant, like the warmth of the sun on your skin, or the coolness of a breeze. It could be something that tastes delicious, like your favorite meal or a healthy snack. You could even focus on a person you care about, an experience of success, or something that causes a positive emotion. For example, you could focus on the smiles on your children's faces, the feeling of being successful at work, or the feeling of being grateful for the good things in your life. To savor, first you focus on the pleasant sight, sound, smell, taste, or touch of the object or event. Next, when you notice positive feelings in your mind or body, you turn your attention inward, and savor the inner feeling, absorbing those positive feelings deep inside yourself like water seeping into soil, and then allowing them to expand. As the positive feelings begin to fade, you return the focus of your attention back to the pleasant object or event, to refresh the positive feelings. And then once again, turn your attention back inward, to savor the inner feeling again. Eventually, you might notice positive memories, associations, or meaningful thoughts arising in your mind. If these come up, you can savor them, too. Shifting your focus back and forth from the outside to the inside and vice versa can deepen and prolong the positive experience, so that you can fully appreciate it. However, no feeling, no matter how positive, can last forever. So once you've deeply savored and appreciated the positive experience, you can feel grateful for it, and let it go.

Let's practice this skill now. Choose one of these savoring objects [**Therapist note**: Let the patient select a flower or stone if you've brought them.] or get the savoring object I asked you to find for your home practice.

[**Therapist note**: You should encourage your clients to select a pleasant, safe, and healthy object for the savoring exercise. If patients forgot to bring an object for savoring practice, or if they are low income and may not have access to a savoring object, you should have extras on hand and supply one. A rose or other flower works great because of its multisensory properties (sight, touch, smell) and associations with love. A piece of fruit, a polished stone, a work of art, or a photograph could also work well. If you are conducting the session over telehealth, the client might choose to savor their pet. Note that when conducting a MORE group, unless you supply the same object of savoring to everyone (e.g., letting them each select a rose from a bouquet), there will be a great variety of objects. To accommodate this variety, you must give very general suggestions during the savoring instruction. These suggestions are detailed in the script below. However, if you have a homogeneous set of savoring objects (e.g., roses), if you like, you could tailor these instructions to be more specific (e.g., "Appreciate the deep red of the rose petals").]

Savoring Practice

You can allow your eyes to close . . . or they can remain open and relaxed on a spot in front of you . . . And you can begin by taking a few mindful breaths . . . Just noticing the natural sensation of the breath . . . Noticing the temperature of that air . . . its warmth or coolness . . . That's right . . . And when the mind is a little more focused . . . a little more settled . . . and a little more open . . . you can open your eyes and begin to focus on the object in front of you . . . Examining it closely, almost as if this were the first time you had ever seen an object like this . . . Appreciating the visual beauty of this object . . . Appreciating the colors . . . The lines and shapes . . . The patterns of light and shadow . . . Really enjoying the beauty of this object . . . And then looking at this object like the way an artist might admire it . . . Softening your gaze . . . Allowing the eyes to relax . . . And take in the object . . . And the space around the object . . . like a single pattern . . . of color, and light, and shadow . . . And soon the space between you and the object may begin to close . . . Sensing a connectedness with the object . . . As if you were becoming one with it . . . That's right . . . And when you notice positive feelings arising in the mind or the body, you can turn your attention inward . . . to savor that pleasant, inner feeling . . . Absorbing those pleasurable feelings . . . Bathing and soaking in the good feelings . . . Savoring that pleasure. . . . Concentrate your attention on these positive emotions and pleasurable sensations, and absorb yourself in those pleasant feelings . . . As if you could breathe in those feelings . . . Breathing them into the center of your being . . . Like water seeping into soil . . . That's right . . .

And then, when you are ready, shifting your attention back to the object . . . And shifting your focus to one of your other senses . . . If the object makes a pleasant sound, appreciating that sound . . . And really taking it in . . . Feeling the sound perhaps like a pleasurable, buzzing sensation . . . If the object has a pleasant scent, appreciating that scent . . . And really taking it in . . . Feeling the scent perhaps like a pleasurable, tingling sensation . . . or touching the object lightly with your fingertips or the skin of your face . . . Appreciating its texture . . . Feeling the sense of contact perhaps like a pleasurable, vibrating sensation . . . Like there was no separation between you and the object . . . Appreciating the life force in this object . . . As if you could breathe in the life force of this object, merging it with your own . . . And when you notice positive feelings arising in the mind or the body, you can turn your attention inward . . . to savor that pleasant, inner feeling . . . Absorbing those pleasurable feelings . . . Bathing and soaking in the good feelings . . . Savoring that pleasure . . . Focus your attention on these positive feelings, and really absorb yourself in them . . . As if you could breathe in those feelings . . . Breathing them into the center of your being . . . Like water seeping into soil . . . That's right . . .

Focusing on these positive feelings, and allowing them to expand and pervade the entire space of awareness . . . With bliss . . . Immersing and infusing awareness with this bliss . . . Now . . . And appreciating the sense of being alive in this moment . . . The gift of life . . . And if the mind begins to wander . . . to meaningful thoughts, or emotions, or memories, or associations with this object . . . That's okay . . . That's what minds do . . . They wander . . . You can just notice what this experience means to you . . . Acknowledging and accepting those thoughts and feelings . . . whatever they are . . . Allowing your mind to expand to include and appreciate these meaningful experiences now . . . That's right . . . Focusing now on the feelings and meanings, allowing them to enrich this experience . . . Holding gratitude for this experience . . . And then, when a deeper part of your mind knows that each time that you practice this it will become easier and easier to savor even more deeply . . . You may feel a little more comfortable, a little more centered, and a little more full of life . . . when you complete this practice.

Process the Savoring Practice (Using PURER)

What did you like best about that experience? Was there anything challenging about it?

People with chronic pain and people in recovery tend to have a lot of suffering. But savoring is a way to self-generate joy and positive emotions, which can help you to cope with pain, be less dependent on opioids to help yourself feel better, and ultimately, enjoy a better quality of life.

To practice savoring, follow these simple steps as described in Handout S4.2:

1. Take a few mindful breaths, or maybe practice a few minutes of mindful breathing.
2. Notice a pleasant object, event, or experience. It could be natural beauty (landscape, mountain, flowers, birds singing in the trees, the warmth of the sun on your skin). It could be an enjoyable physical movement or exercise. It could be the taste of a healthy meal. It could be the sense of connection with a loved one or a friend. It could be a sense of accomplishment, safety, or satisfaction.

3. Pay attention to the sights, sounds, smells, textures, and temperature of the object or experience.
4. Pay attention to how your body feels in response to the pleasant event. Pay attention to how your mind responds to the pleasant event.
5. When you notice positive feelings in the mind or body, or positive thoughts or memories in response to the pleasant event, focus on those positive feelings and thoughts and allow them to deepen and grow stronger. Then imagine as if you could breathe in and absorb those positive feelings "like water seeping into soil."
6. If the mind wanders to distractions, pain, or negative thoughts or feelings, accept those thoughts and feelings, let them go, and gently return your focus back to the pleasant object, event, or experience.

Home Practice

- Review Handout S4.2. Savoring
- Daily mindfulness-of-pain or body scan practice
- Daily reappraisal practice (with Handout S3.2)
- Daily savoring practice
- STOP (Handout S1.5)

Common Pitfalls, Troubleshooting, and Closing Advice for the Therapist

Note that some objects of savoring carry complex emotional associations. For instance, once a participant in MORE savored a rose and began to cry. His mother, whom he loved, grew roses in her backyard. The client's mother had died, and so savoring brought up powerful feelings of affection and grief, simultaneously. Be prepared to process these complex emotions with PURER. Get phenomenological to identify how the client used mindfulness to become aware of and accept the complex emotional experience. Reframe sadness as an indication of the meaning and poignancy of the object and its associations. Provide education that mindfully savoring emotions, even difficult ones, can help the patient to "digest" the feeling and move on from it. Provide reinforcement around the notion that the patient has the courage to face difficult feelings while still appreciating the beauty of the object and the memories it carries. And ask the client how they can use what they have learned from this experience of savoring, in spite of, or perhaps because of, the powerful emotions that it evoked.

When we are experiencing pain or something stressful, that painful or stressful event becomes the center of our focus, and we ignore the parts of our life that are positive or maybe not so bad. We become laser focused on the painful or stressful thing—it's a kind of tunnel vision. That painful or stressful thing becomes the sole focus of our awareness—it's all we see.

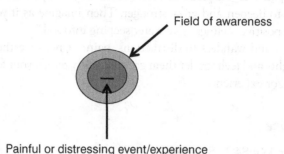

Field of awareness

Painful or distressing event/experience

The tunnel vision of attentional bias.

But we can learn to use mindfulness to zoom out from this tunnel vision, and expand the field of our awareness to encompass not only the painful or distressing parts of life but also the many neural and positive events and experiences that occur on a daily basis. Mindfulness gets us out of the tunnel by expanding our vision. And then we can begin to practice savoring by noticing and appreciating the positive aspects of our life. And when we do that, the painful parts of our life become smaller by comparison. The negative things can still be there, but they are no longer a central focus. They can start to fade into the background.

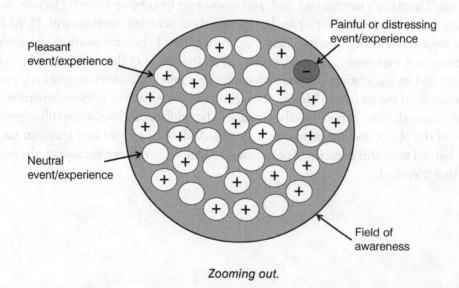

Painful or distressing event/experience

Pleasant event/experience

Neutral event/experience

Field of awareness

Zooming out.

Handout S4.2. Savoring

Savoring is a way to increase positive feelings, and to enjoy your life more deeply. It's a simple practice, but also extremely powerful and important. To savor, first notice a pleasant object, event, or experience. For example, you could savor natural beauty (e.g., a flower or sunset), delicious healthy food, the sense of connection (e.g., the feel of your child's hand), or even an accomplishment (e.g., a project you completed successfully). Then use that experience as the object of your mindfulness practice.

Begin with a few minutes of mindful breathing. Then, when your mind is more focused and more open, focus your attention on the pleasant features of the object/event/experience. Appreciate the pleasant colors, shapes, and lines. Appreciate the patterns of light and shadow. Look at the object almost as how an artist would look at it. Allow your gaze to relax and take in the whole object along with its background, like one whole pattern of color, shape, light, and shadow. Notice how the distance between yourself and the object might begin to close, and feel a sense of closeness, interconnectedness, or oneness with the object.

Next, notice if there are sounds. What do you hear? Is there really a separation between yourself and the sound? Notice your other senses. What do you smell? What do you taste? What do you touch?

Then, notice any positive emotions or pleasant body sensations that come up during the practice. When you notice positive emotions (e.g., happiness, joy, excitement, calm) or pleasant sensations (e.g., warmth, tingling, energy, bliss), turn your attention inward and appreciate and absorb the positive emotions and pleasurable sensations that arise in your mind and your body. When the positive feeling fades, return your attention back to the pleasant object/event/experience to savor it some more. When you notice positive feelings, turn your attention inward again, to savor the positive inner feeling. Toggle back and forth between savoring the pleasant things you sense in the object/event/experience and the positive feelings arising inside of you.

Eventually, become aware of the life force in the object. Recognize your own life force. Appreciate the sense of being alive in this moment. If your mind wanders to meaningful thoughts, memories, or associations, that's okay, that's what minds do, they wander. Acknowledge and appreciate where the mind has wandered off to. Maybe it has something to teach you. Finally, take a few long moments to savor the best parts of the experience. Rest your mind in whatever positive feelings have been generated from this practice.

Session 5

Mindfulness as Freedom
from Craving

Agenda

Mindfulness-of-pain practice: 22 minutes

Process in-session mindfulness-of-pain practice (using PURER): 7 minutes

Process mindfulness home practice and STOP (using PURER): 8 minutes

Process reappraisal home practice (using PURER): 5 minutes

Process savoring home practice (using PURER): 10 minutes

Break: 10 minutes

Opioid dependence and craving: 20 minutes

Mindfulness-of-urges practice: 25 minutes

Process mindfulness-of-urges practice (using PURER) 10 minutes

Assignment: 3 minutes—discuss and assign for the following week:

- Daily mindfulness of pain or body scan
- Daily reappraisal
- Daily savoring
- STOP

Materials Needed

Chocolate or other candy for each group member

Paper towels to wipe hands clean

Handout S5.1. Mindfulness of Urges

Session Introduction for the Therapist

This session is one of the most important, and challenging, of the MORE program. Here, you will introduce the concept of craving, a very contentious subject among people who are prescribed opioids for pain. Many such patients have an implicit or explicit belief that if opioids are being used to relieve pain, then there will be no craving—that craving is something only "addicts" experience. In fact, patients on long-term opioid therapy do sometimes experience craving, but it is often conflated with the desire for pain relief—that is, patients often believe they are feeling the need to take opioids to alleviate their pain, but in actuality, their urge to take opioids is being driven by unconscious appetitive impulses (e.g., craving) or opioid withdrawal as the last dose wears off. Because *craving* is such a loaded term, here you will lean more heavily on the term *urge for opioids*, which tends to be perceived more neutrally. The wording in this section has been carefully constructed to not offend patients, but nevertheless therapists should be mindful that some patients may take offense at the words and concepts discussed. Be prepared to apologize or rescind any of your statements that create resistance. You can give the disclaimer "What I'm about to talk about may not fit your situation perfectly."

The session culminates in the mindfulness-of-urges technique, which expands upon the "candy exercise" in Session 2 by teaching the use of mindfulness to zoom in to craving as a means of deconstructing it, coupled with the use of reappraisal as a means of contemplating the consequences of opioid dependence. Note that this technique is long and complex, and may evoke strong feelings. Make sure to leave an adequate amount of time to process the mindfulness-of-urges exercise so that patients do not leave the session with escalated levels of craving or distress.

Session Script

Mindfulness-of-Pain Practice

Use the practice on pages 100–101 in Session 2.

Process the In-Session Mindfulness-of-Pain Practice (Using PURER)

What did you like best about that experience? Was there anything challenging about it?

Process the Mindfulness Home Practice

How did you use mindfulness this week to help yourself with pain, opioid use (or addiction recovery)?

[**Therapist note:** The question about addiction recovery should only be asked if the group is comprised of people with OUD in recovery.]

Process the STOP Practice

When you were focused on your breathing, what did you notice about your attention for the medication/drug? Did it keep getting pulled back to the medication/drug? What did you notice in your body when your attention was focused on the medication/drug? What thoughts did you notice? What did you do when you noticed your attention was captured by the medication/drug? Did you notice that you could bring your attention back to your breath, and keep it there longer? Did you find that you were more disinterested in the medication/drug, like you didn't care that much about it? Were you able to "step back" or practice "zooming out" during this experience? And were you able to use mindfulness, reappraisal, and savoring skills to manage difficult feelings instead of relying on opioids?

Process the Reappraisal Home Practice

How did you use reappraisal this week to help yourself with stress, opioid use (or addiction recovery)?

[Therapist note: The question about addiction recovery should only be asked if the group is comprised of people with OUD in recovery.]

Process the Savoring Home Practice

How did you use savoring this week to help yourself feel better or appreciate life more?

Opioid Dependence and Craving

Today, we will spend time talking about opioid medications, like oxycodone, hydrocodone, and morphine. As we discussed in the first session, there is a lot of stigma in our society around opioids.

Have you ever felt stigmatized by your use of opioids?

This stigma can make it hard to talk about issues and problems related to taking opioids. In the short term, opioid use can alleviate pain. Yet, there are many side effects of taking opioids, and over the long term, they may not only become less effective in controlling pain but also can negatively impact your overall health. But I'm not here to tell you that opioids are bad or to push you to stop taking them. Instead, the goal of this program is to provide you with another tool to help deal with pain that has no negative side effects. Mindfulness can actually improve your health!

When a person takes opioid pain medication frequently over months or years their body and brain can become so used to the medication that it may become less effective over time. When this happens, the person's ability to deal with pain may decrease, and so they may feel that they need to take higher doses of opioids just to feel okay. This is called tolerance. Tolerance is one side effect of long-term opioid use, and is a sign of physical dependence on opioids. Another sign of dependence and a side effect of long-term opioid use is withdrawal. This means that if you have been taking opioids for a long time, your body and brain are so used to having the opioids on board that if you stop taking them all at once, your nervous system becomes imbalanced, which can make you feel sick and all sorts of other uncomfortable sensations. If you stop the pills cold turkey, you could experience flu-like symptoms, cramps, nausea, stomach pain, diarrhea, headaches, body aches, sweating or flushing, goosebumps, anxiety, depression, or irritability.

Have you ever experienced tolerance or withdrawal? What was it like for you?

There are many other side effects to taking opioids over the long term. Opioids can cause constipation, bowel problems, vomiting, drowsiness, difficulty concentrating, and dizziness. Less commonly, opioids can impair your immune system and have negative effects on your hormone levels. Also, long-term opioid use can in some cases cause hyperalgesia—an increase in pain levels. Research has shown that taking opioids over an extended period of time can increase the sensitivity of your nervous system to pain. This could cause your original injury to hurt worse over time, or other parts of the body that used to not hurt might start hurting.

Many people who take long-term opioids don't even notice this is happening to them. They think their pain condition is getting worse, so they assume that they should take a higher dose of opioids to alleviate the pain. But taking more opioids just fuels a vicious cycle. Taking more opioids can make the brain and body more sensitive to pain, and so the person takes an even higher dose. This becomes a downward spiral of opioid dependence.

Also, sometimes people take opioids to get relief from emotional pain, like stress, depression, anger, or anxiety. Sometimes people discover this by coincidence. They take an opioid for pain, but then they discover in the process that it also makes them feel better emotionally, too. It chills them out. For some people when they take opioids it's like all of their emotional problems go away in an instant. Some people have said that the first time they took opioids was the first time in their life when they felt at peace or a sense of well-being. So, in the short run, opioids can relieve emotional pain in addition to physical pain.

Can you relate to this idea in some way?

Research shows that in the long run, for some people opioids can actually make them moodier over time. Long-term opioid use can make you more sensitive to stress, irritation, depression, and anxiety.

Using opioids for reasons other than physical pain (like to relieve emotional distress), or taking them in higher doses than prescribed, is called opioid misuse. While most people who take opioids do not misuse them, misuse is also not uncommon—some studies suggest that as many as a quarter of people with chronic pain on long-term opioids misuse them from time to time. To be clear, misuse is not addiction. Misuse just means taking opioids differently from how they were prescribed. But opioid misuse can lead to a fatal overdose, and it can also lead to addiction.

Regardless of whether they misuse opioids, some people like the feeling of taking opioids, and some people don't. Even if you don't like the way opioids make you feel, sometimes you might feel a strong need or urge to take the medication. You might feel an urge to get some relief, or an urge to make yourself feel better.

Is urge the right word to describe this? What about craving? What words would you use?

Most people agree that they want to take the medication to get relief, and they feel that they *must* take it, even if they don't like taking opioids. This kind of ambivalence can become an intense internal struggle.

Have you ever felt conflicted about taking opioids?

Just as we talked about automatic pain-coping habits, the urge to use opioids can become a habit, too. You may not be able to relate to this at all, but some people experience this. Most patients are told to take opioid medication on a schedule to prevent the pain from getting worse. But when you do this, this might turn opioid use into a habit. As we discussed in Session 2, the automatic habit of opioid use has triggers. People who have become dependent on opioids can have triggers that set off the urge to take a pill. Triggers can be a time of day, a place, a feeling of pain, a feeling of stress or negative emotions, or other events, objects, or people that activate the urge to use opioids. For example, if you keep your pills in the medicine cabinet in your bathroom, when you open the medicine cabinet, that might trigger the urge to take a pill. For many people struggling with opioid-related problems and dependence, emotional pain and stress can be powerful triggers.

What are some of your automatic triggers for the urge to use opioids?

These thoughts of taking opioids or urges can pop up often, and can occupy a lot of your time. They can fill your mind and intrude into your day. These thoughts can interfere with your social life, your family, and your work. When they occur frequently or intensely, they can become very distressing. It can become difficult to resist or turn away from these thoughts. It can be very difficult to stop or control them.

Have you ever had this experience? How did you react to it?

If you feel a strong need or urge to take your medication, but you don't take it because you've run out of medication, you forgot your pills at home, or you have decided to start reducing your dose, you might start to notice uncomfortable sensations in your body and difficult emotions in your mind. People usually think that these urges and uncomfortable feelings are their body telling them that they *must* take more medication. But this is not necessarily true. Really, these feelings are a side effect of the body and brain getting used to functioning with less opioids.

Sometimes people take opioids to get relief from these urges and uncomfortable feelings. But if you try to escape these feelings by taking another dose of opioids, your dependence on opioids will deepen, and the urges and uncomfortable feelings will grow stronger.

On the other hand, if you experience the urge to take more opioids but you only take as much medication as your doctor prescribed, or even try to taper down your dose under your doctor's guidance by gradually increasing the time between doses or skipping "as-needed" doses that you don't really need, the urges will become weaker and eventually fade away. Urges, like pain sensations, come and go over time. How long does an urge last if you don't give into it? If you feel the urge to take an opioid but you choose to not take it, it can be an interesting experiment to see just how long the urge lasts before it fades away on its own.

Just like you've learned to use mindfulness to deal with pain, you can also use mindfulness to deal with urges. You can learn to use mindfulness to cope when you want to take opioids, but you can't because you ran out, don't want to take more than prescribed, or are in recovery and no longer using opioids.

Mindfulness of Urges

Unfortunately, the pain-relieving effects of opioids may last only so long. If you are trying to spread out your doses to make them last, you may notice physical discomfort, stress, and anxiety during the time in between doses. Or, sometimes you may be in a situation when you don't want to take a pill. Let's say you are going out to a dinner party with friends, and you don't want to feel groggy or out of it from your pills. But if you skip a dose, not only might you feel discomfort but you might find it hard to stop thinking about opioids.

There are effective ways to use mindfulness to counteract the uncomfortable thoughts and feelings that come up with the need or urge for opioids.

One mindfulness technique involves zooming in to the urge to break it down, just like you've learned to zoom in to pain. Just like pain, an *urge* is just a word we use to describe a mix of sensations, thoughts, and feelings. When you use mindfulness to zoom in to an urge, you will discover that the *thing* that you called an urge is actually many things: your heart beating faster, your mouth filling up with saliva, a feeling of jitteriness or emptiness in the pit of your stomach, the muscles of your neck and shoulders getting tighter, your palms getting sweaty, or the image of yourself about to take a pill. As you continue to use mindfulness to zoom in to the urge, you will notice that these sensations and images might start to change as time passes. Your fast heartbeat might start to slow down, and your muscle tension might become a tingling, or a sense of vibration, or energy. When you zoom in, you can discover that the urge is something that changes from moment to moment, and as you break it down into its parts, dealing with any of those thoughts or sensations might be easier than dealing with the overwhelming experience of the urge as a whole. Eventually, you might notice that the urge is fading away or becoming less intense so that you don't even care that much about it anymore. You don't have to react to it. Intensely focusing your mindful awareness on the urge can help you to pierce through it, like using a magnifying glass to focus the sunlight into a white-hot point that is so intense it can burn a hole through a leaf or a piece of paper. Focusing mindfulness on the urge can cause it to evaporate, just like the rays of the sun can evaporate a drop of water.

Another mindfulness technique for dealing with urges involves contemplating the reasons why you want to learn how to live without being dependent on opioids. This is a kind of reappraisal.

What are some of the reasons why you want to reduce your dependence on opioids? What will you gain from learning how to cope with pain by taking less opioids or by being less dependent on opioids? How will your life be better?

If you notice an urge for opioids coming up, you can first use mindfulness to step back from that urge. Then, you can begin to think deeply about the reasons why you want to become less dependent on opioids. This might be especially hard to do on those days when your pain is really bad, or maybe when you are really stressed out. On days like that, the urge to take opioids might be really strong. Of course, you know in the back of your mind the reasons why you want to learn to live without being dependent on opioids. If you didn't, you probably wouldn't be in this group right now. But that knowledge is more powerful when you move it from the back of your mind to the front of your mind. When you consciously contemplate and call to mind the reasons why you want to learn to manage pain with less medication, and how your life could be better when you are less dependent on opioids, the urge will become weaker. If you find that your mind starts to wander back to the urge, you can use mindfulness to refocus back on the reasons why you want to become less dependent on opioids, again and again. And each time that you do this, you will become more determined. Your strength of will becomes stronger.

The mindfulness-of-urges technique I'm about to teach you combines both of these approaches—zooming in to the urge and contemplating reasons to use less medication—to strengthen your self-control over your opioid use. If you've ever felt out of control when it comes to your pain or opioid use, strengthening your self-control can be empowering. Mindfulness of urges is a form of mental training. It builds the muscle of your self-control. Let's practice this form of training now. We will practice with the candy exercise that we did in the second week's session. However, this time, I will ask you to imagine that you are holding opioids in your hand. Try to use mindfulness to cope with any urges that come up, and notice how your experience of urge differs this time from the first time you did this exercise.

Mindfulness-of-Urges Practice

[Therapist note: Use chocolate or another kind of candy.]

Sitting comfortably but regally, as if you were a king or queen, or perhaps as if you are a warrior about to go into battle . . . With spine straight and belly relaxed . . . You can begin by practicing a few moments of mindful breathing . . . Just noticing the natural sensation of the breath . . . Noticing the temperature of that air . . . its warmth or coolness . . . That's right . . . Just noticing the natural sensation of the breath . . . And then, when the mind is a little more focused . . . a little more centered . . . a little more open . . . You can allow your eyes to open . . . And focus your attention on the piece of candy in your hand . . .

If the chocolate has a wrapper . . . You can slowly unwrap it . . . But don't eat it yet! . . . Once unwrapped, you can hold the chocolate up before your eyes . . . Paying close attention to it . . . Noticing its color . . . Its texture . . . And as you turn the chocolate slowly to look at it from different angles, perhaps noticing how the sugar crystals glint in the light . . . That's right . . .

Next, bring the chocolate up to your nose, and smell it . . . Notice its delicious scent . . . You can become aware of the exact moment when you feel the urge to eat it, but don't eat it yet . . . And we have this word urge, but what is it really? . . . Zooming in to those sensations now . . . Perhaps the smell of the chocolate makes your mouth fill with saliva . . . Perhaps noticing sensations of hunger . . . Jitteriness? . . . Heat? . . . Heaviness? . . . Tightness? . . . Tingling? . . . Emptiness? . . . Are there thoughts or feelings associated with those sensations? . . . And can you notice if the sensations have a center? . . . Can you notice if they have edges? . . . Perhaps the sensations are not solid . . . Perhaps there are spaces inside the sensation, where the sensation is not . . . Observe what it is like to have an urge to eat chocolate but to not give in to that urge . . .

And if the sensations become too intense . . . You can notice where the uncomfortable sensations are not . . . You can focus on the feeling of the air moving into the tip of your nostrils as you breathe . . . You can always return your attention back to the breath . . . As a way to recenter yourself . . . As a way to zoom out from sensation . . . And now imagine that you can breathe right into those intense sensations . . . Imagining that you can send your breath right into those sensations, breathing into the sensations, to soften them, like water seeping into soil . . . That's right . . . And then, return the focus of your attention back to the sensations . . . Can you notice how they are changing? . . . Perhaps the intensity is changing . . . Perhaps gradually getting weaker? Perhaps becoming more intense, reaching a peak, and then gradually getting weaker? . . . Perhaps the quality of the sensation is changing . . . Can that jitteriness become a warmth? . . . Can the tightness become tingling? . . . An emptiness become a sense of energy? . . . Or vibration? . . . Or a spaciousness? . . . Perhaps the location is changing . . . You can notice if the sensations have a center . . . You can notice if they have edges . . . Perhaps the sensation is not solid . . . Perhaps there are spaces inside the sensation, where the sensation is not . . . And then you can let those sensations go, and gently but firmly return the focus of the attention back to the breathing . . . That's right . . .

Now, imagine that instead of holding that chocolate, you are holding an opioid in your hand . . . You can see the opioid just a few inches from your face . . . You can see its color, what it looks like . . . You might think about how your body feels when your opioids kick in . . . That's right . . . You may begin to notice an urge soon, even as a part of you begins to really want to take those opioids . . . And we have this word urge, but what is it really? Zooming in to those sensations now . . . Perhaps noticing sensations of jitteriness . . . Heat? . . . Heart beating faster? . . . Sweating . . . Heaviness? . . . Tightness? . . . Tingling? . . . Emptiness? . . . Are there thoughts or feelings associated with those sensations? . . . Thoughts like "Why can't I have this?" or "What's wrong with me that I want this?" . . . Perhaps an image of yourself about to take an opioid . . . And can you notice if the sensations have a center? . . . Can you notice if they have edges? . . . Perhaps the sensations are not solid . . . Perhaps there are spaces inside the sensation, where the sensation is not . . . Observe what it is like to have an urge to take opioids but to not give in to that urge . . .

And if the sensations become too intense . . . You can notice where the uncomfortable sensations are not . . . You can focus on the feeling of the air moving into the tip of your nostrils as you breathe . . . You can always return your attention back to the breath . . . As a way to recenter yourself . . . As a way to zoom out from the sensations . . . And now imagine that you can breathe right into those intense *sensations . . . Imagining that you can send your breath right into those sensations, breathing into the sensations, to soften them, like water seeping into soil . . . That's right . . . And then, return the focus of your attention back to the sensations . . . Can you notice how they are changing? . . . Perhaps the intensity is changing . . . Perhaps gradually getting weaker? . . . Perhaps becoming more intense, reaching a peak, and then gradually getting weaker? . . . Perhaps the quality of the sensation is changing . . . Can that jitteriness become a warmth? . . . Can the tightness become tingling? . . . An emptiness become a sense of energy? . . . Or vibration? . . . Or a spaciousness? . . . Perhaps the location is changing . . . you can notice if the sensations have a center . . . You can notice if they have edges . . . Perhaps the sensation is not solid . . . Perhaps there are spaces inside the sensation, where the sensation is not . . . And then you can let those sensations go, and return your attention back to the breath . . . That's right . . .*

Now you can take a few long moments to consciously contemplate the reasons why you want to become free from dependence on opioids . . . You can deeply focus on the reasons why you really want to learn how to cope with pain by taking less opioids . . . You can think about the negative consequences of being dependent on opioids, how being dependent on them has hurt you . . . and hurt the people you love . . . Then, you can think about how your life will be better when you are less dependent on opioids . . . How freeing yourself from opioid dependence will help you . . . and help the people that you love . . . And if you notice positive feelings arising in the mind or the body, you can savor those positive feelings now . . . That's right . . . And then you can let those thoughts and feelings go . . . And return your attention back to the breath . . .

And each time that you notice that the mind has wandered to thoughts or feelings or urges . . . And you become aware of where the mind has wandered off to . . . And you acknowledge and accept that thought and feeling . . . And then you return the focus of your attention back to the reasons why you want to become freer from opioids . . . You are learning to step back . . . to step back . . . to step back from your urges and into the clear, open space of mindfulness . . . You are strengthening your mindfulness . . .

And soon you may begin to notice that urges, thoughts, and feelings come and go on their own, like clouds passing in a clear blue sky . . . Like clouds drifting, urges come out of nowhere, gradually change shape . . . And then fade into the distance, all on their own . . . And there is no need to hold them or to push them away . . . You can just let them go . . . And a part of the mind is like those urges passing like clouds . . . But there is a deeper part of the mind . . . that is more like . . . the space in which the clouds pass . . . the observing awareness . . . that is open . . . spotless . . . stainless . . . and free . . . Just watching, just observing . . . peacefully . . . And you can focus your attention on that part of your mind, or you can continue to focus your attention on the breath . . . That's right . . . And now, you can take a few long moments to focus on the best parts of this experience . . . Appreciating and savoring whatever positive feelings or thoughts have come up for you during this practice . . . or you can continue to focus on the breath . . . And when you know that each time you practice this, it will become easier and easier to use mindfulness to free yourself from urges . . . You may feel a little more comfortable . . . A little more centered . . . And a little more empowered . . . When you open your eyes and return your attention to the room.

Finally, return your attention to the chocolate. You can choose to eat the chocolate, or to throw away the chocolate now, as a symbol of the power you have to make choices over what you put in your body.

[**Therapist note**: Put a trash can in the center of the group so patients can throw away the chocolate. This can be a powerful ritual and symbol. However, the therapist should eat the chocolate, to send an implicit message of nonjudgment and that patients will not be shamed for future opioid use.]

Process the Mindfulness of Craving Practice (Using PURER)

What did you like best about that experience? Was there anything challenging about it?

Now that you have learned how to use mindfulness to deal with urges, you can use this tool whenever you need to. This technique is described in Handout S5.1. If you are interested in reducing your opioid use, the mindfulness of urges technique could help you to deal with any uncomfortable feelings that come up when you start cutting down your opioid doses. If you are working to overcome opioid addiction or are in addiction recovery, this technique can help you to get through cravings and prevent yourself from slipping back into the habit of drug use. You can practice this technique anytime you need to manage the urge to take opioids (or other substances, including alcohol or unhealthy food).

Home Practice

- Review Handout S5.1
- Daily mindfulness-of-pain or body scan practice
- Daily reappraisal practice (with Handout S3.2)
- Daily savoring practice
- STOP (Handout S1.5)

Common Pitfalls, Troubleshooting, and Closing Advice for the Therapist

If working with patients with opioid misuse and/or OUD, you should assess craving by the end of the session. If craving levels remain high, offer an additional 5- to 10-minute mindful breathing practice (like the practice in Session 1) as a way to de-escalate patients before ending the session. Patients could be triggered by this technique, so it is important to assess for safety and provide de-escalation as needed through mindfulness or other techniques like reappraisal, relaxation therapy (Wright et al., 2017), or motivational interviewing (Miller & Rollnick, 2023) to prevent relapse. Although you should remain aware of the possibility that this technique might prompt intense cravings that remain unresolved by the end of the treatment session, in prior research studies of MORE, no adverse events related to this technique have been noted.

Handout S5.1. Mindfulness of Urges

An urge (also known as a craving) is a strong desire, want, or need. Sometimes when people take opioids over an extended period of time, they can develop urges to take the medication. When you are taking opioids on a schedule, you might not even notice any urges. But if you aren't able to take opioids because you've run out of medication, you forgot your pills at home, or you have decided to start reducing your dose, you might begin noticing uncomfortable sensations in the body and difficult emotions in the mind. Sometimes people take opioids to get relief from these urges and uncomfortable feelings. However, urges don't last forever. They will fade away on their own, if you don't give into them. But if you try to escape these feelings by taking another dose of opioids, your dependence on opioids will deepen, and the urges and uncomfortable feelings will grow stronger. On the other hand, if you experience the urge to take more opioids but you only take as much medication as your doctor prescribed, or even try to taper down your dose under your doctor's guidance by gradually increasing the time between doses or skipping "as-needed" doses that you don't really need, the urges will become weaker and eventually fade away. You can use mindfulness to deal with urges.

When you want to use mindfulness to overcome urges, you can sit down and practice the full mindfulness-of-pain practice, which takes about 15–20 minutes to complete. In this practice, you begin with a few minutes of mindful breathing. Then, when your mind is a little calmer and more focused, focus your awareness on the urge itself. Remember, *urge* is just a word, but what is it really? Use your attention to "zoom in" to the experience of the urge, and break it down in to sensations of tightness, or jitteriness, or hunger, or other sensations. Notice if there are thoughts or feelings associated with those sensations. Then notice if the sensations have a center. Notice if they have edges. Notice if there are spaces inside the sensation where the sensation is not. Maybe the sensation is not solid. If the sensation becomes too intense, refocus your attention on your breathing as a way to "zoom out" from the sensation of the urge. Then imagine as if you could send the breath into the sensations, to soften them, like water seeping into soil. And then zoom back in to the sensations and notice how they are changing over time. Perhaps the intensity is changing (getting weaker, or first getting stronger and then getting weaker). Perhaps the quality of the sensations is changing. And notice if the sensations have a center. Notice if they have edges. Notice the spaces inside the sensation where there's no sensation at all.

Now, return your attention back to your breath for a few breaths, and then take a few long moments to consciously contemplate the reasons why you want to free yourself from this urge.

Think about the negative consequences of indulging in the urge, and how indulging in this urge has hurt you and the people you love. Think about the positive consequences of freeing yourself from the urge, and how freeing yourself from this urge will help you and the people you love.

Then, let those thoughts go. Notice how you can "step back" or "zoom out" from your thoughts and sensations to observe them like a witness. Notice how sensations, like thoughts, come and go, all on their own, like clouds passing in a clear blue sky. Become aware of the space in which the clouds pass, the observing awareness, that is open, spotless, stainless, and free, just watching and observing, peacefully. Rest your awareness on that part of your mind. Finally, take a few long moments to savor whatever positive feelings you have generated from this practice.

Session 6

Breaking the Chain between Emotional Pain and Craving

Agenda

Mindfulness-of-pain practice: 27 minutes

Process in-session mindfulness-of-pain practice (using PURER): 7 minutes

Process mindfulness home practice and STOP (using PURER): 8 minutes

Process reappraisal home practice (using PURER): 5 minutes

Process savoring home practice (using PURER): 10 minutes

Break: 10 minutes

The stress reaction and the mindful response to stress: 10 minutes

Imaginal stress exposure: 5 minutes

Mindful relaxation response practice: 10 minutes

Process imaginal stress exposure exercise (using PURER): 8 minutes

Body scan practice: 12 minutes

Process body scan practice (using PURER): 5 minutes

Assignment: 3 minutes—discuss and assign for the following week:

- Daily mindfulness of pain or body scan
- Daily reappraisal
- Daily savoring
- STOP

Materials Needed

Handout S6.1. Mindful Relaxation Response

Session Introduction for the Therapist

This session is relatively light on psychoeducational content. Instead, the session centers around three extensive mind–body techniques (mindfulness of pain, mindful relaxation response, and body scan). The mindful relaxation response technique is included in case there are participants still struggling with the core skill of mindfulness by Session 6. This technique, involving slow breathing and imagery, is more concrete than the mindfulness-of-pain technique, and therefore may be more accessible to participants who have struggled to grasp mindfulness, which relies on higher-order cognitive functions of attention regulation and meta-awareness.

Session Script

Mindfulness-of-Pain Practice

Use the practice on pages 100–101 in Session 2.

Process the Mindfulness of Pain Practice (Using PURER)

What did you like best about that experience? Was there anything challenging about it?

Process the Mindfulness Home Practice (Using PURER)

How did you use mindfulness this week to help yourself with pain, opioid use (or addiction recovery)?

[**Therapist note:** The question about addiction recovery should only be asked if the group is comprised of people with OUD in recovery.]

Process the STOP Practice

When you were focused on your breathing, what did you notice about your attention for the medication/drug? Did it keep getting pulled back to the medication/drug? What did you notice in your body when your attention was focused on the medication/drug? What thoughts did you notice? What did you do when you noticed your attention was captured by the medication/drug? Did you notice that you could bring your attention back to your breath, and keep it there longer? Did you find that you were more disinterested in the medication/drug, like you just didn't care about it? Were you able to "step back" or practice "zooming out" during this experience? And were you able to use mindfulness, reappraisal, and savoring skills to manage pain and difficult feelings instead of relying on opioids?

Process the Reappraisal Home Practice

How did you use reappraisal this week to help yourself with stress, opioid use (or addiction recovery)?

[**Therapist note:** The question about addiction recovery should only be asked if the group is comprised of people with OUD in recovery.]

Process the Savoring Home Practice

How did you use savoring this week to help yourself feel better or appreciate life more?

The Stress Reaction and the Mindful Response to Stress

Life can be stressful. Though sometimes stress seems to hit you all at once, like a freight train, the stress process is actually made up of several stages that unfold really fast, within just a few seconds. The first stage is when we experience the stressful event. That's the *activating event* that we talked about in the *ABCDE* model in Session 3. Maybe someone yells at you, or you get a huge bill in the mail that you weren't expecting, or get in a fender bender with your car. During the next stage, your brain makes a rapid determination to figure out whether the event represents a present danger, or whether it is something that might hurt you in the near future. I'm not just talking about physical danger here, but also, the event might harm you by causing you to lose something that really matters to you, like your financial security, your good reputation, or even the people you care about. This determination is called a *stress appraisal*. Remember the term *reappraisal* from Session 3? If you make the appraisal that the event might be harmful, then the next stage in the stress process occurs. During this next stage, you determine whether you have what it takes to solve the problem or cope with the stressor. These appraisals can happen within a second or two. They happen so fast that we often don't notice them. Our mind just sizes up the situation for us, automatically and unconsciously. That's why you sometimes walk into a situation and get a *bad feeling*, maybe a churning in your gut or the hair starts to stand up on your neck. If you determine that you can't handle the event and solve the problem, the next stage of the stress process happens. You start to experience the consequences of stress. You might start to feel overwhelmed or anxious. Your heart begins to beat faster, your palms become sweaty, and muscles get tight.

When someone with chronic pain experiences the tight muscles that come with stress, what do you think it does to their pain?

People who suffer from chronic pain can experience a flare-up of pain in response to stress and other forms of emotional pain like depression, anxiety, resentment, and anger. There are several reasons for this. When you are stressed, your muscles get tight, and these tight muscles can add to back, neck, shoulder, and jaw pain. Also, when you are stressed, your heart beats harder, it pumps more blood to your head and brain, and this can bring on a headache or make it worse. In addition, stress can increase inflammation in the body, and inflammation can really aggravate chronic pain. Stress can even make your gut hurt; when you are stressed, your brain sends signals to your stomach and intestines, which can cause cramps, bloating, nausea, diarrhea, or constipation. But, most importantly, when you are stressed, your brain turns up the volume of the sensations from the body. Stress can make a minor injury hurt way worse. Remember how we talked about how the brain can turn the volume of your pain up and down? Well, stress jacks that volume way up.

And, if you are someone who takes opioids to deal with pain, or if you are in recovery from opioid addiction, stress can lead to powerful urges for opioids.

Can you tell me about a time when you noticed that stress increased your urge to take opioids?

Sometimes people take opioids when they are feeling stressed, depressed, worried, ashamed, guilty, or angry. If you have developed the habit of taking opioids to make yourself feel better emotionally, and you are in a stressful or upsetting situation, the experience of emotional pain can increase the urge to take opioids. Also, being stressed can make it harder to control your habits. Have you ever heard the expression "He pushed my buttons"? When we use that phrase, we are referring to the fact that stress can actually trigger automatic habits. We call that the stress reaction. This is the final stage of the stress process.

But the stress reaction isn't inevitable. There's another, healthier way of dealing with stress. We can respond mindfully to the stressors in our lives. Mindfully responding to stress involves being conscious of the stress process, starting with the stress appraisal. We can reevaluate our interpretation of the stressful event and our ability to cope with it. We can do that through reappraisal—the *ABCDE* technique you learned in Session 3. What's the proof that the event is really harmful? What's the proof that it's not harmful? What's the proof that you can't handle it? What's the proof that you can handle it? Think back to the other stressful times in your life. Remember how you coped with them successfully in the past, and overcame them. Remind yourself of your strengths, your skills, and your capabilities. Then ask yourself: What's a more helpful way of thinking about this situation? If you had a friend in this situation, what would you want them to believe? How will going through this tough time make you a stronger person? How can it teach you something or help you to grow? These questions can help calm down your mind and help you to deal with the stressor more effectively.

Though reappraisal is a great way to reduce stressful thoughts, your body might still feel stress in the form of the symptoms we talked about earlier (e.g., tension, fast heartbeat, sweating). To deal with the uncomfortable symptoms of stress in the body, you can use a mindful relaxation response. This skill involves some slow, focused breathing, and the use of your imagination. To learn how to use this skill when you really need it, first I will ask you to imagine being in a stressful situation . . . maybe something stressful that happened to you this week. If there was a stress scale from 0 to 10, with 0 being no stress whatsoever, and 10 being the most stressed you've ever been, pick a situation that's about a 3 on that scale. Once you imagine being stressed, I will guide you through the mindful relaxation response to reduce that stress.

[**Therapist note:** Use a fast-paced and staccato urgent voice tone during the imaginal stress exposure. Model the stress in your own face and body. Use the opposite approach to *soothing the baby* that you use in normal mindfulness instruction. Startle the baby! Then, when you get to the mindful relaxation response section, shift to a soothing voice tone and slow pacing, to suggest relaxation and calm.]

Imaginal Stress Exposure

[**Therapist note:** Use fast, staccato voice and pacing.]

Allow your mind to wander back to that situation when you felt stressed . . . Remember what was happening in this stressful situation . . . Imagine where you were when this stressful situation happened . . . You can imagine the people involved in the situation . . . You can see their faces . . . You can hear their voice tone, you can hear what they are saying . . . You can imagine what is happening in this situation that is stressing you out . . . The difficult things, the hassles, the problems . . . The things that cause you concern . . . Soon you can imagine feeling that stress in your body . . . Your muscles are becoming tight . . . Can you feel the tension in your lower back? . . . Your neck and shoulders? . . . All over the body? . . . Can you feel your heart beating faster, your increased blood pressure? . . . Maybe you are breathing faster . . . Short, shallow breaths . . . Can you feel yourself sweating? . . . Can you notice feelings of jitteriness or worry? Imagining yourself getting really stressed out now . . . And as the feeling of stress grows stronger in your body, you might even start to notice an urge to take opioids . . . But you can remember . . . You can experience stress and urges, but you don't have to react to them . . .

Mindful Relaxation Response Practice

[**Therapist note:** Use slow, soothing voice and pacing.]

Now, let those stressful thoughts and feelings go . . . And return the focus of your attention to your breath . . . Breathing deeply and slowly, allowing your breath to fill up the lungs . . . Breathing into your belly . . . Breathing in for a count of 3 . . . 1, 2, 3 . . . Holding it for a count of 3 . . . 1, 2, 3 . . . and breathing out for a count of 3 . . . 1, 2, 3 . . . Breathing in for a count of 3 . . . 1, 2, 3 . . . Holding it for a count of 3 . . . 1, 2, 3 . . . and breathing out for a count of 3 . . . 1, 2, 3 . . . Breathing in . . . Holding it . . . Breathing out . . . Breathing in . . . Holding it . . . Breathing out . . . Breathing in . . . Holding it . . . Breathing out . . . That's right . . .

And with each passing breath . . . You can imagine a warm, colored light, any color that you like, flowing into the body . . . Imagining breathing in this warm colored light, any color that you like . . . That's right . . . A warm, healing light . . . Breathing that light into your heart, into the center of your being . . . And imagining that healing, colored light filling up the body, almost as if the body were like a pitcher of water, and you were filling it up with water . . . With each passing breath . . . Breathing in that warm colored light, any color that you like . . . Filling up the body, flowing up an axis along your spine . . . And breathing out that warm colored light, out the top of your head, like a beam shining high up into space above you . . . Allowing your mind and awareness to float up into space . . . And spreading outward . . . Like the branches of a tree . . . That's right . . .

And now as you breathe out, imagine that any stress or craving or discomfort is flowing out of the body . . . Like a black thread spiraling down . . . Down through the head . . . Down the neck . . . Down the chest . . . Down the abdomen . . . Down the legs . . . Down through the feet . . . Down through the floor . . . Down into the center of the earth . . . Spreading like the roots of a tree . . . Spreading down until it is many miles below, settling deeply in the earth . . . Releasing any stress or craving . . . Purifying the mind and body . . . Breath relaxing, muscles relaxing, body relaxing . . .

Then again, breathing in that colored light . . . And imagining that healing, colored light filling up the body, as if the body were a pitcher, and you were filling the pitcher up with water . . . Breathing in that warm colored light, any color that you like . . . Filling up the body . . . Allowing that warm, healing light, any color that you like, to completely fill the space of the whole body . . . The whole body . . . The whole body . . . And then imagining that light shining out beyond the body . . . Into space . . . As if you were like the sun . . . Light radiating into space . . . Until the space inside the body, and the space outside the body . . . are one space . . . Resting the mind in that space, now . . .

And when you are ready, you can complete this practice . . . Allowing your eyes to open . . .

Process the Mindful Relaxation Response (Using PURER)

What did you like best about that experience? Was there anything challenging about it?

You can practice this technique on your own by following the instructions in Handout S6.1.

Body Scan Practice

The body scan is another powerful practice that can be used to reduce the impact of stress on the body. You learned the body scan in Session 1 as a way to understand the concept of mindfulness. But now you can use the body scan to produce a powerful mindful relaxation response.

Sitting comfortably . . . You can allow your eyes to close . . . or they can remain open and relaxed on a spot in front of you . . . You can begin by bringing your attention to the top of the head, to the scalp, just noticing the sensations there, whatever they are . . . And then letting them go . . . Moving the attention down to the forehead, just noticing the sensations there . . . whatever they are . . . And then letting them go . . . Moving the attention down to the muscles around the eyes, and the eyes themselves, just noticing the sensations there . . . whatever they are . . . And then letting them go . . . Moving attention to the inside of the head, to the center of the head, to the brain, just noticing those sensations there . . . whatever they are . . . And then letting them go . . . Moving the attention down to the jaw, the mouth, the lips, the teeth, the tongue, just noticing those sensations there . . . whatever they are . . . And then letting them go . . . Moving the attention down to the neck and the shoulders, just noticing the sensations there . . . whatever they are . . . And then letting them go . . . Moving the attention to the chest, to the heart, just noticing those sensations . . . whatever they are . . . And then letting them go . . . Moving the attention down the arms, to the hands, just noticing the sensations there . . . And then letting them go . . . Moving the attention to the abdomen, to a point right behind your belly button, at the center of your being, just noticing the sensations there . . . And then letting them go . . . Moving the attention to the low back, just noticing the sensations there . . . And then, letting those sensations go . . . Moving the attention to the hips, to the pelvis, just noticing sensations there . . . whatever they are . . . And then letting them go . . . Moving the attention to the thighs, just noticing the sensations there . . . whatever they are . . . And then letting them go . . . Moving the attention down to the knees, to the lower legs, to the calves, just noticing the sensations there . . . whatever they are . . . And then letting them go . . . Moving the attention to the feet, to the toes, just noticing the sensations there . . . And then letting them go . . . Then sweeping the attention as if it were a spotlight or a flashlight through the body . . . From the tips of the toes, to the top of the head . . . And from the top of the head, to the tips of the toes . . . From the front of the body to the back . . . And back to the front . . . From the inside, to the outside . . . And from the outside to the inside . . . Then, expand the attention to encompass the whole body, becoming aware of the whole body, the whole body, the whole body . . . Then, perhaps becoming aware of the sensations a few inches in the space beyond the body, like the sensations in the space just above your head . . . Then perhaps becoming aware of the space near the ceiling . . . In the corner of the room . . . Then perhaps becoming aware of the space above the ceiling, above the building . . . The space of the sky . . . And then perhaps becoming aware of the space beyond the sky . . . Out in space . . . Toward the center of the galaxy . . . The center of the universe . . . Resting your mind in that space now . . . or continuing to focus on sensations in the body . . . That's right . . . And now you can take one long moment to focus on the best part of this experience . . . Appreciating and savoring any positive experiences that have come up during this practice . . . Then, when a deeper part of your mind knows that each time that you practice this, it will become easier and easier to go even more deeply into the state of mindfulness . . . You may feel a little more comfortable, a little more centered, and a little more at peace . . . When you complete this practice and bring your attention back to the room.

Process the Body Scan (Using PURER)

What did you like best about that experience? Was there anything challenging about it?

Home Practice

- Review Handout S6.1
- Daily mindfulness-of-pain or body scan practice
- Daily reappraisal practice (with Handout S3.2)
- Daily savoring practice
- STOP (Handout 1.5)

Common Pitfalls, Troubleshooting, and Closing Advice for the Therapist

For the imaginal stress exposure exercise, be sure to have patients select a stressful situation that is about a 3 on a scale of 0–10. Don't open up a can of worms you can't put back together again. This note of caution is particularly important in this session, as unlike during the reappraisal practice in Session 3, here you will not be processing the patient's stressor. If, during PURER processing of this exercise, a patient expresses difficulty engaging the mindful relaxation response to a particularly traumatic stressor, you might have to help guide them with reappraisal to address maladaptive cognitions associated with this stressor event. However, in general, these types of difficulty rarely arise in this session, and most patients find themselves very relaxed by the completion of the body scan—the third mind–body technique in this session.

Handout S6.1. Mindful Relaxation Response

Stress can make chronic pain and opioid use worse. We can reduce stress by first using mindfulness to step back from stressful thoughts and then by using reappraisal to change our negative thoughts about the stressful life situation. But sometimes even after using reappraisal our bodies still might feel stressed out (e.g., muscle tension, fast heartbeat, sweating). To deal with the uncomfortable symptoms of stress in the body, you can use a mindful relaxation response. This skill involves some slow, focused breathing, and the use of your imagination.

Begin by sitting or lying down with your eyes closed. First breathe in for a count of 3. Then hold your breath for a count of 3. Then breathe out for a count of 3. Continue this slow breathing for about 10 breaths. Then, imagine breathing in a warm, colored light, any color that you like. Imagine that this light is a healing light. Imagine breathing it into your heart, into the center of your being. Imagine that healing, colored light filling up the body, almost as if the body were like a pitcher of water, and you were filling it up with water. Imagine that healing, colored light filling up the body, flowing up your spine. Then imagine breathing the warm, colored light out of the top of your head, like a beam shining high up into space above you. Allow your mind and awareness to float up into space and spread outward like the branches of a tree.

Next, as you breathe out, imagine that any stress or craving or discomfort is flowing out of the body like a black thread spiraling down through the head, neck, chest, abdomen, legs, and feet. Imagine the stress, craving, or discomfort spreading down through the floor, and down to the center of the earth, spreading like the roots of a tree. Release any stress or craving. Relax the body.

Finally, imagine breathing in that healing, colored light, allowing it to completely fill the space of the whole body. And then imagine that light shining out beyond the body, into space, as if you were like the sun. Experience the space inside the body, and outside the body, as one space, and rest your mind in that space for as long as you like.

Session 7

Mindfulness to Meaning through Interdependence

Agenda

Mindfulness-of-pain practice: 32 minutes

Process in-session mindfulness-of-pain practice (using PURER): 5 minutes

Process mindfulness home practice and STOP (using PURER): 5 minutes

Process reappraisal home practice (using PURER): 5 minutes

Process savoring home practice (using PURER): 5 minutes

Break: 10 minutes

Interdependence as the middle way between dependence and independence: 20 minutes

Meditation on interdependence practice: 15 minutes

Process meditation on interdependence practice (using PURER): 10 minutes

Reflection on recovery and meaning in life: 10 minutes

Assignment: 3 minutes—discuss and assign for the following week:
- Daily mindfulness of pain or body scan
- Daily reappraisal
- Daily savoring
- STOP

Materials Needed

Raisins, fresh fruit, or vegetables

Handout S7.1. Mindfulness to Meaning and Interdependence

Session Introduction for the Therapist

Unlike previous sessions that largely focus on symptom reduction, this session is focused on help-ing patients to cultivate a sense of meaning in life and through awareness of interdependence, to experience self-transcendence: the sense of being connected to something greater than the self. In MORE, the concept of interdependence is heavily influenced by the Buddhist doctrine of *pratītyasamutpāda*—codependent arising—which acknowledges that all phenomena are depen-dent on causes and conditions and therefore lack an individual, independent existence (Rahula, 2007). This session, with its psychoeducational material and a meditation on interdependence, has a decidedly philosophical, existential, and spiritual focus. In this sense, MORE goes beyond the cognitive-behavioral tradition by fully embracing positive psychology's emphasis on centering eudaimonic meaning and self-actualization within the scope of psychotherapy.

Eliciting meaning and self-transcendence via the concept of interdependence may help patients who are deeply identified with their chronic pain to recognize that their true identity transcends pain. Here we also discuss the possibility of becoming attached to or dependent on opi-oids, and that addiction can become part of one's identity. As in many other places throughout the eight sessions, if you anticipate that you will encounter strong resistance around concepts related to addiction, or are working with patients who take opioids as prescribed by their physicians, you might omit or modify this material to be more palatable or appropriate.

Session Script

Mindfulness-of-Pain Practice

Use the practice on pages 100–101 in Session 2.

Process the Mindfulness of Pain Practice (Using PURER)

What did you like best about that experience? Was there anything challenging about it?

Process the Mindfulness Home Practice

How did you use mindfulness this week to help yourself with pain, opioid use (or addiction recovery)?

[**Therapist note:** The question about addiction recovery should only be asked if the group is com-prised of people with OUD in recovery.]

Process the STOP Practice

When you were focused on your breathing, what did you notice about your attention for the medication/drug? Did it keep getting pulled back to the medication/drug? What did you notice in your body when your attention was focused on the medication/drug? What thoughts did you notice? What did you do when you noticed your attention was captured by the medication/drug? Did you notice that you could bring your attention back to your breath, and keep it there longer? Did you find that you were more disinterested in the medication/drug, like you just didn't care about it? Were you able to "step back" or practice "zooming out" during this experience? And were you able to use mindfulness, reappraisal, and savoring skills to manage pain and difficult feelings instead of relying on opioids?

Process the Reappraisal Home Practice

How did you use reappraisal this week to help yourself with stress, opioid use (or addiction recovery)?

[**Therapist note:** The question about addiction recovery should only be asked if the group is comprised of people with OUD in recovery.]

Process the Savoring Home Practice

How did you use savoring this week to help yourself feel better or appreciate life more?

Interdependence as the Middle Way between Dependence and Independence

In this program you've learned to use mindfulness to zoom in to and zoom out from pain, stress, and opioid dependence. But mindfulness can be used to zoom out even farther than that. We can learn to use mindfulness to get a bird's-eye view on our lives, to see our lives from a broader perspective. When we do that, we can start to appreciate what is truly important and meaningful in life.

Usually the things in life that we want the most become what's most important to us. Some things that many people want include love, money, success, or fun and excitement. But, when we start to want something bad enough, we become dependent on it—attached to it. We start to believe that we can only feel truly happy if we have that thing, or that relationship. Without it, we believe that life has no meaning. This approach to life is a problem, because nothing lasts forever. Everything changes over time. So, the more we come to want something, the more attached we get, and then when that thing fades away, we feel a deep sense of pain and loss. When we become attached like that, things that used to make us feel good become a trap—a form of dependence.

Taking opioids can become that same kind of thing: a form of dependence. Many people become physically dependent on opioids, or psychologically dependent on them. Even if you don't like how opioids make you feel, even if you don't want to take them, over time you might come to feel like you must have them just to feel okay, just to be able to feel like yourself and function normally. When opioid dependence progresses to addiction, sometimes people start to feel like their whole lives revolve around opioids: craving them, thinking about where to get them, and worrying about what will happen when they run out. When opioid use progresses to this point, the people, activities, and values in life that the person once found meaningful become less important, as more and more time and energy becomes focused on obtaining and using opioids.

People can even become dependent on their pain—not because they want to feel pain but because they start to feel defined by it. I know that might sound strange. But, over time, chronic pain may feel like it's become part of your identity—part of who you are as a person. Every time you visit with a new doctor, you have to tell the story of your pain, when it started, what it's like, how it affects your life, and the things you've tried to make it better—again and again. You might feel like pain has stolen the things from you that you care about the most—maybe you can't do the things you used to love to do. Maybe you say no to social engagements because going out hurts too much, maybe you can't help out around the house as much as your spouse or partner needs, maybe you can't pick up your kids and grandkids to give them a hug. Maybe many of the things you used to do—that defined you—seem like they have been taken away from you by pain. Instead of thinking of yourself as a great homemaker, or a hard worker, or a professional, or an athlete, now maybe you just think of yourself as someone with chronic pain. Instead of spending time doing the things you care about doing, maybe you find yourself spending more and more time going to medical appointments, trying to find a solution to your pain. You might start feeling like your whole life is wrapped up in your pain.

How has your identity seemed defined by your pain or opioid use?

Dependence isn't the only problematic approach to life. Having too much independence can also be an issue. We usually think independence is a great thing. They say no man is an island, but some of us try to live that way anyway. Sometimes when people think they should be independent, they feel like they don't need anyone, and that no one can or should help them. This approach can lead to social isolation and loneliness. People might start to think that they should be able to rise above the problems in their life, all on their own. They might reject help when it is offered to them for fear of appearing weak. But if that happens too many times, there won't be help available when they need it. Someone who is trying to be independent might want to push past their problems and sweep them under the rug, to get them behind them and just move on. One way that people try to get past the things they don't like, like feelings of sadness, anger, or anxiety, is to try to push those feelings away. But, when you try to brush off difficult thoughts and feelings, to ignore and suppress them, sometimes they just come back stronger. For example, have you ever noticed that if you feel really angry about something that happened to you, and you don't want to think about it, the more you try to get it out of your head, the more it comes back to you? Suppression doesn't work in the long run—it can backfire and make things worse.

But there is an alternative to falling into the trap of too much dependence or independence. This alternative approach involves zooming out to acknowledge and accept difficult thoughts and feelings as important pieces of the larger whole of your life, and to recognize that who you truly are is much bigger than any one thought or feeling. Who you really are is much bigger than any single part of your life. We've been hinting at this in every mindfulness exercise, especially when we talk about observing thoughts, feelings, and sensations like clouds passing in a clear sky. There's a part of yourself that is like those thoughts and feelings, passing like clouds. But there is a deeper part of yourself that is more like the space in which the clouds pass: a space large enough to contain all clouds, but a space beyond them, totally clear and cloudless, full of light.

Instead of trying to push away unwanted experiences, and instead of craving and dependence, there is an alternative perspective you can take. You can take a bird's-eye view and broaden your focus to see how everything that happens in your life has its own meaning or purpose; everything that arises can be a teacher—even the painful parts of life. This way of seeing is called interdependence.

Here's a simple example of interdependence from nature. Animals and plants are interdependent on each other to live. To survive, animals need to breathe oxygen, and plants need to breathe carbon dioxide. When an animal breathes, it inhales oxygen, and exhales carbon dioxide. When a plant breathes, it takes in carbon dioxide, and then releases oxygen back into the air. Animals breathe in the oxygen that the plants breathe out, and plants breathe in the carbon dioxide that animals breathe out. In this very physical way, animals and plants are totally interdependent. But, in addition to needing carbon dioxide, plants also need to grow in nutrient-rich soil. In the forest, when a tree branch breaks and falls to the ground, and when plants and animals die, their material gets broken down in the soil and their matter becomes compost and fertilizer to provide nutrients to other plans and animals. In other words, even hurts and losses can have a purpose or meaning.

Why am I telling you this? When we begin to expand our awareness beyond the anger and the sadness that often comes with having chronic pain or being dependent on opioids, we can begin to see how we are deeply interconnected to something greater than ourselves. In the forest, this greater whole is evident. Everything in the forest fits together perfectly; every aspect of life has its niche. The oaks shade the fungus, the fungus decomposes the bark, the bark feeds a beetle, that feeds a bird, and the bird feeds your heart by filling your ear with the beauty of its song. So everything has its purpose; everything happens for a reason. And as you realize this, the question of the meaning of life may come into focus, and you can begin to see how everything that has ever happened to you has shaped you and made you into the person you are today.

In other words, every breath we take and every action we do affects the world around us, and in return, everything that happens in the world has an impact on us. Think about the people close to you, and how much you have been affected by your parents, your spouse, your children, your teachers, and your friends. You literally would not exist if your parents had never met each other. Would you really be the same person that you are today if you never had all of the important experiences that you had with people you care about? Would you be the same person you are today if you had never met these people in the first place? Now, recognize how much your actions have affected others. We are as independent with one another as are the animals and plants in the forest. All living things take part in this great web of interdependence. Because all beings are dependent on one another for their existence, and because everything in life is interdependent, everyone and everything has a purpose or meaning. Even going through the difficult parts of life, like physical pain, emotional suffering, problems with opioids, or addiction, may have a purpose or a meaning. Painful life experiences may have something important to teach you. Sometimes people come to realize that facing chronic pain and illness has actually helped them to develop inner strength or made them wiser, more appreciative, more grateful, and more compassionate to the suffering of others. In this way, adversity can actually teach us something really important and provide a path toward spiritual growth.

What are some ways you can relate to this idea? Can you tell me about a time in the past when you had to face something difficult in life, and facing that challenge helped you to grow as a person?

When you use mindfulness to zoom all the way out to take a bird's-eye view on your life, you can see the big picture, how all the pieces of your life fit together into one great puzzle, one great pattern. Everything that happens has its rightful place. Even the difficult things in life taught you something and shaped you into the person you are today. When you take this broader perspective, you can come to see life's challenges as potential sources of personal growth and meaning. And you can appreciate and savor the many joys and gifts you have been given. The joy and the pain are also interdependent, all tied together into one single whole, into the story of your life. This deep sense of interdependence—this sense of being connected to something greater than yourself—can be a powerful focus for mindfulness practice. We will now do a mindfulness exercise to experience this, and then have a discussion afterward.

[**Therapist note**: Hand out a raisin to each group member, or if the patient is participating in a telehealth session at home, they could use whatever fruit or vegetable is available. If patients use different types of fruits or vegetables, it can get tricky, but try to provide general suggestions that cover all classes of fruits and vegetables—for example, "You can see the leaves of the plant on which this fruit or vegetable grew."]

Meditation on Interdependence Practice[1]

Sitting comfortably, but with grace, as if you are a wise sage remembering some deep and important wisdom . . . You can allow your eyes to close . . . or they can remain open and relaxed on a spot in front of you . . . And then take a few mindful breaths . . . Noticing the sensation of the breath moving into the nostrils . . . Noticing the warmth or coolness of that air . . . That's right . . . And soon you may notice that the mind begins to wander . . . And if the mind wanders, that's okay, because that is what minds do—they wander . . . Just noticing where the mind has wandered off to . . . acknowledging . . . and accepting that thought or feeling . . . And then, you can let it go . . . And then gently, but firmly, bring the attention back to the sensation of the breath moving into the nostrils . . .

When the mind is a little more focused, a little more centered, and a little more open . . . You can allow your eyes to open . . . And then shift the attention to the raisin in your hand . . . You can observe this raisin as if you had never seen a raisin before . . . As if it were the first time you had ever seen an object like this . . . Observe its color . . . its shape . . . its texture . . . Peer deeply at this object, as if you could use your eyes to zoom in to it . . . Almost as if you could see the tiny particles it is made of . . . Seeing deeply into the nature of this object . . .

And as you do this . . . Imagine that you can see through the raisin, through time and space . . . Can you see this raisin as a grape growing on a vine? . . . You can see the color of the vine . . . The vibrant green of its leaves . . . Absorbing the sunlight . . . You can see the vine rooted in the dark, rich earth . . . Full of compost . . . Watered by the rain, cooled by the breeze . . . Growing more and more with each passing moment . . . And each passing day . . . Growing many bunches of grapes . . . Ripening in the sun . . . And then you can imagine how people came and picked the grapes . . . So the grapes could dry into raisins . . . People working hard, feeling tired and sore from all the hard work . . . Then workers came and loaded them into boxes . . . And loaded those boxes onto trucks . . . Straining under the heavy burden . . . Backs aching . . . For a purpose . . . Then drivers drove those trucks hour after hour, day after day, until they reached their destination . . . At the store . . . Where the raisins were bought . . . And now . . . Sometime later . . . A raisin rests in your hand . . .

Peering deeply into that raisin, can you see the bunch of grapes from which it came? . . . Can you see the green of the leaves, the woody stem of the vine? . . . Can you see the dark richness of the soil? . . . Can you see the insects, birds, and small animals that fertilized the soil and turned it into rich compost? . . . Can you imagine each of their lives? . . . Can you feel the warmth of the sun on your skin? . . . Can you feel the coolness of a breeze? . . . Can you feel the cool, cool rain? Can you see the hands of the workers, and feel the ache in their bodies? . . . Can you see how every person, every plant, every piece of dirt is born from the earth? . . . Did you know that the earth long ago was born out of the sun? . . . So every piece of dirt, every molecule, every atom that makes up everything you see was born in the heart of a star . . . So the raisin is the star . . . The star is in that raisin . . . Can you see it? . . .

Then, when you are deeply focused, deeply absorbed . . . Place the raisin in your mouth . . . And slowly chew the raisin, but don't swallow it . . . Savoring its favor . . . Can you can taste everything that came together to create this raisin? . . . The purple grapes? . . . The green leaves . . . The woody vine . . . The rich dark soil . . . The compost . . . The nourishing rain . . . The coolness of the breeze . . . The warmth of the sun . . . Allow the raisin to melt and dissolve into your mouth . . . And as this raisin

[1] From *Mindfulness-Oriented Recovery Enhancement for Addiction, Stress, and Pain* by Eric L. Garland. Copyright © 2013 NASW Press. Adapted by permission of the National Association of Social Workers.

dissolves into you, the grape . . . the leaves . . . the vine . . . the soil . . . the compost . . . the rain . . . the breeze . . . the workers . . . their burden . . . the earth . . . the sun . . . and the stars are becoming one with you . . . One taste . . . Savoring this one taste . . . Of existence . . . Of just being, in the moment . . . Savoring the flavor of life . . . The taste of being alive, in this moment . . . The taste of your connection with everything . . . And when you finally swallow, know that all things are a part of you, just as you are a part of them . . . Savoring this sense of interdependence, this sense of oneness . . . now . . . And then, when you are ready, bringing your attention back to the room.

Process the Meditation on Interdependence Practice (Using PURER)

What did you like best about that experience? Was there anything challenging about it?

Reflection on Recovery and Meaning in Life

Throughout this program, you have been learning skills to strengthen your recovery from chronic pain (and addiction). Recovery has been defined as a "deeply personal, unique process of changing one's attitudes, values, feelings, goals, skills, and/or roles. It is a way of living a satisfying, hopeful, and contributing life even with limitations caused by illness [pain, or addiction]. Recovery involves the development of new meaning and purpose in one's life" (Anthony, 1993, p. 11).

Reflecting now on everything we just talked about and experienced, if someone were to ask you what the meaning of your life is, what would you tell them? How has dealing with your pain (and addiction) helped you to develop new meaning, taught you something important, made you more compassionate, or helped you to grow as a person? What is the meaning of your recovery from pain (and addiction)? How can recovery bring a sense of meaning to your life? How can knowing what makes life meaningful to you help to stay motivated to continue your recovery journey?

I encourage you to reflect on the rich discussion we just had and complete Handout S7.1 sometime after group finishes today so you can really reflect on and remember your sense of meaning and purpose in life.

Home Practice

- Review and complete Handout S7.1
- Daily mindfulness-of-pain or body scan practice
- Daily reappraisal practice (with Handout S3.2)
- Daily savoring practice
- STOP (Handout 1.5)

Common Pitfalls, Troubleshooting, and Closing Advice for the Therapist

Note: This is the most abstract and spiritual session in the MORE program, and often, the most meaningful. Patients often report that this is the first time they had ever considered their interdependence with others and the world around them. When doing the meditation on interdependence, using any fruit or vegetable will work. It doesn't have to be a raisin. If you use a different fruit/vegetable, tailor the language in the script to match the growing/harvesting process of that fruit/vegetable. In processing both the first mindfulness meditation of the session and the meditation on interdependence, keep your ears open for reports of self-transcendence, of the participant connecting with something greater than the self. Patients might report a deep quieting of the mind, feelings of spacious expansiveness beyond the body, an experience of pure being, or oneness. Get phenomenological and delve into those reports, and provide a hearty dose of positive reinforcement around them. Finally, make sure to save plenty of time at the end of the session to hold the discussion about recovery and meaning in life.

In the MORE program you've learned to use mindfulness to zoom in to and zoom out from pain, stress, and opioid dependence. But mindfulness can be used to zoom out even more than that. We can learn to use mindfulness to get a bird's-eye view on our lives and to see our lives from a broader perspective. When we do that, we can start to appreciate what is truly important and meaningful in life. From a bird's-eye view, you can broaden your focus to see how everything that happens in your life has its own meaning or purpose; everything that arises can be a teacher—even the painful parts of life. This way of seeing is called interdependence.

To become mindful of interdependence, focus deeply on one part of your life or your experience, something that you think is significant, or perhaps even something that you assume isn't very significant. Think back to the raisin exercise that we did in Session 7. You could use that same way of seeing with other objects and events in your life. Look deeply at that object or event and contemplate where it comes from: its origin. Contemplate the many steps and stages it had to go through in order to show up in your life at this moment. Contemplate the many other factors that affected this object or event and made it what it is today. Contemplate how it has affected and continues to affect you and the people you are close to. Contemplate what this object and event means to you, now and for your future. In doing this, you will have a sense of its meaning. You will see that the object or event doesn't exist by and for itself; it exists as part of an interdependent network.

A final and important step is to reflect on how you also exist as part of an interdependent network, and how you too have meaning. Reflect on the meaning of your recovery.

Throughout this program, you have been learning skills to strengthen your recovery from chronic pain (and if this is an issue for you, recovery from addiction). Recovery has been defined as a "deeply personal, unique process of changing one's attitudes, values, feelings, goals, skills, and/or roles. It is a way of living a satisfying, hopeful, and contributing life even with limitations caused by illness [pain, or addiction]. Recovery involves the development of new meaning and purpose in one's life" (Anthony, 1993, p. 11).

Contemplate this meaning and purpose by reflecting on and writing about the topics on the blank worksheet on the next page.

(cont.)

Reflecting on your recovery and what you have learned in the MORE program, if someone were to ask you what the meaning of your life is, what would you tell them?

How has dealing with pain or opioid-related issues helped you to develop new meaning, taught you something important, or made you grow as a person?

What is the meaning of your recovery from pain (and if this is an issue for you, recovery from addiction)? How can recovery bring a sense of meaning to your life?

How can knowing what makes life meaningful to you help you stay motivated to continue your recovery journey?

Session 8

Maintaining Mindful Recovery

Agenda

Mindfulness-of-pain practice: 40 minutes

Process in-session mindfulness-of-pain practice (using PURER): 5 minutes

Process mindfulness home practice and STOP (using PURER): 5 minutes

Process reappraisal home practice (using PURER): 5 minutes

Process savoring home practice (using PURER): 5 minutes

Break: 10 minutes

Reflecting on what you have learned: 10 minutes

Designing an effective mindful recovery plan: 20 minutes

Future pacing with imagery rehearsal practice: 10 minutes

Process future pacing with imagery rehearsal (using PURER): 7 minutes

Closing: 3 minutes

Materials Needed

Handout S8.1. Mindful Recovery Plan

Session Introduction for the Therapist

This final session presents the longest meditation practice of the program. Remember to inject long periods of silence between suggestions (and particularly, in the space between complex suggestions). If you notice clients with facial expressions indicating strong emotions or difficulty, you can "throw them a lifeline" with your voice, giving them a suggestion like

"And now you can notice where your mind is in this moment . . . Is it focused on the breath? . . . Or lost in thoughts and feelings? . . . Perhaps even strong feelings . . . But wherever the mind is, that's okay . . . You can just notice where the mind is in this moment . . . Acknowledge and accept that thought or feeling . . . Let it go, and return the focus of the attention back to the breath."

Then, you can drop back into silence. Later in the session, you will discuss the concept of recovery and guide the clients to develop a recovery plan. Note that the word *recovery* is now a loaded term and widely associated with addiction. If you are working with clients who do not identify with being addicted, this term might create some discomfort. To counter this issue, give a general definition of the term that is as applicable to chronic pain as it is to addiction. As in the previous sessions, be mindful to omit or modify language like "addiction," "craving," and "triggers" if you believe it will be stigmatizing or is inappropriate to the particular clients in your group (e.g., the group members do not misuse opioids or have an OUD).

Session Script

Today we start with the longest mindfulness practice of this program. You've strengthened your mindfulness so much over the past 7 weeks, I know you are ready for a deep practice. So let's begin.

Mindfulness-of-Pain Practice

Use the practice on pages 100–101 in Session 2.

Process the In-Session Mindfulness-of-Pain Practice

What did you like best about that experience? Was there anything challenging about it?

Process the Mindfulness Home Practice

How did you use mindfulness this week to help yourself with pain, opioid use (or addiction recovery)?

[Therapist note: The question about addiction recovery should only be asked if the group is comprised of people with OUD in recovery.]

Process the STOP Practice

When you were focused on your breathing, what did you notice about your attention for the medication/drug? Did it keep getting pulled back to the medication/drug? What did you notice in your body when your attention was focused on the medication/drug? What thoughts did you notice? What did you do when you noticed your attention was captured by the medication/drug? Did you notice that you could bring your attention back to your breath, and keep it there longer? Did you find that you were more disinterested in the medication/drug, like you didn't care as much about it? Were you able to "step back" or practice "zooming out" during this experience?

And were you able to use mindfulness, reappraisal, and savoring skills to manage pain and difficult feelings instead of relying on opioids?

Process the Reappraisal Home Practice

How did you use reappraisal this week to help yourself with stress, opioid use (or addiction recovery)?

[**Therapist note:** The question about addiction recovery should only be asked if the group is comprised of people with OUD in recovery.]

Process the Savoring Home Practice

How did you use savoring this week to help yourself feel better or appreciate life more?

Reflection on What You Have Learned

This program has been all about strengthening recovery. Recovery has been defined as "a process of change through which individuals improve their health and wellness, live a self-directed life, and strive to reach their full potential" (SAMHSA, 2012). This program is founded on the idea that recovery from chronic pain, opioid-related problems, and addiction is possible. You can recover and reclaim a meaningful life from pain, emotional distress, and addiction.

What have you learned from this program that can help you strengthen your recovery in the future?

You've spent the last 8 weeks in the MORE program learning mindfulness, reappraisal, and savoring skills to help you to cope with pain with less medication, to use the power of your own mind to relieve pain and stress, and to live a more meaningful life. You've come a really long way, but there will still be challenges in the future. Let's take some time to come up with a plan for how you can use what you have learned from this program to strengthen your recovery.

Designing an Effective Mindful Recovery Plan

It's important to have a plan of what to do when things get tough. Without a plan, stressors can start to pile up fast and the next thing you know, you may feel totally overwhelmed. It might seem like it's impossible to get your pain or opioid use under control again. But if you have a plan of how you can address challenges as they arise, when problems occur things won't completely fall apart. You can tackle them head on, and be proactive instead of reactive. Let's use the Mindful Recovery Plan worksheet (Handout S8.1) to write down your plan. There are five important steps to coming up with a mindful recovery plan:

1. Identifying your triggers
2. Identifying strategies to address each trigger
3. Identifying a plan to continue your mindfulness practice
4. Identifying what you can do if you experience a lapse
5. Identifying your reasons for recovery

Let's walk through each of these steps, and as we do so, write down your recovery plan on the worksheet.

[**Therapist note**: Pass out Handout S8.1 with pens/pencils and have participants complete this worksheet as you discuss each item.]

First, think about what might trigger a bad flare-up of pain in the future. Then think about what might trigger you to increase your opioid use. To figure this out, reflect on your past experiences.

In the past, when you experienced bad pain flare-ups or significant increases in opioid use, what kinds of things were happening in your life at those times? What activating events, beliefs/ thoughts, emotions, or people may have triggered you?

Write those down in Section 1. Next, consider the mindfulness, reappraisal, and savoring skills you have learned in this program.

How can you use what you have learned to manage triggers, stress, pain flare-ups, and the urge to take more opioids?

In Section 2, write down, next to each trigger, how you will cope with it by using one of the skills you have learned in this program.

The next time one of these triggers shows up in your life, what specific actions will you take to deal with it?

You've been practicing mindfulness, reappraisal, and savoring skills for the past several weeks. By now, your skills are getting pretty strong. But, remember: This is a "use it or lose it" situation. If you don't practice your skills regularly, your mindfulness muscle will get out of shape. The best way to keep your mindfulness strong is to practice your skills on a regular basis. You want to hardwire your mindfulness practice into a positive habit, so that it just becomes a part of you. Scheduling your practice at the same time of day can help. Setting reminders on your phone or computer can help. Asking family members to encourage you or hold you accountable is another way to keep up your practice. Or, you could join a meditation group to help encourage you to practice. You could even connect with the members of this group to support one another in your practice.

How will you continue your regular practice of mindfulness, reappraisal, and savoring on your own? When will you practice? What days and times? How can you remind yourself to practice? How can you stay motivated to practice? Which people in your life can support you and encourage you to practice?

Write down the answers to these questions in Section 3. Next, it is important to consider what you will do if you lapse back into old, negative automatic habits. Through this program you may have cut down on your opioid use or managed to come off opioids completely. You might be functioning better and being more active in your life, in spite of pain. But it's possible that in the future, you might experience some new pain or stressor, and find yourself taking opioids again or taking opioids in higher doses than you were prescribed. You might find yourself becoming less active. Maintaining a commitment to the positive changes you've made can be a two-steps-forward, one-step-back kind of process. But if you stick with it, you will eventually get many steps ahead toward your goal. Many people slip back to old habits several times before ultimately changing their habits.

Those who successfully change negative habits and ultimately lay them to rest learn from their mistakes and use those learnings to ensure their success.

Instead of thinking, "Now that I've blown my progress, everything is over. I might as well just forget it, and go back to my old way of dealing with things," what would be a more helpful way of thinking about a lapse? If you do have a lapse, what steps can you take to resume your recovery plan?

Write down the answers to these questions in Section 4. Last, it's important to identify your reasons for recovery. You've been working very hard the past several weeks to help yourself change and grow. Why is recovery important to you? Consider the people you care about, the activities you find meaningful, and your deepest values and aspirations. Once you've identified your reasons for recovery, you can commit time and energy to these things. When you pursue the activities that really matter to you, when you connect with the people who you really care about, and when you savor the beauty all around you, the meaning of your life will grow, and pain, opioids, and stress will become smaller by comparison. You will have committed yourself to a recovery-oriented way of life.

What are your reasons for recovery? What motivated you to start this program, and to stick with it? Who are the important people in your life? What kind of a person do you really want to be? What are your values? What actions do you need to do, and what ideas do you need to hold on to, to live a meaningful life, and to live your life the way you want to live?

Write down the answers to these questions in Section 5.

Now, to bring all of these ideas together, we end by doing a practice of imagining yourself in the future—successful, strong, and wise—using the skills you've learned to live your life the way you want to live. Doing so will give you a clear picture of where this recovery journey is leading. Once you've seen the goal, and the path it takes to get there, you will be motivated to take the steps you need to take to achieve what you want to achieve.

Future Pacing with Imagery Rehearsal Practice

You can begin with a few mindful breaths . . . Noticing the sensation of the breath moving into the nostrils . . . Noticing the warmth or the coolness of that air . . . Just noticing the natural sensation of the breath . . . That's right . . . And even as a part of your mind becomes more focused on the breath in this moment . . . You can allow another part of your mind to begin to drift . . . More like a mind floating in space . . . More like a mind floating in time . . . To a moment, in the not too distant future, when you have achieved what you want to achieve and are now living your life the way you want to live . . . Soon you can imagine yourself in this moment . . . Like a character on a movie screen . . . You can see what you are doing in this moment that shows . . . You have achieved what it is that you want to achieve, and are now living your life the way you want to live . . . You can see your body, your posture, the way that you are moving that shows . . . You have achieved what it is that you want to achieve, and are now living your life the way you want to live . . . You can see your expression, the look on your face, the look in your eyes that shows . . . You have already achieved what it is that you want to achieve, and are now living your life the way you want to live . . . And when you see your eyes in that moment . . . You can go through those eyes, deep inside of yourself . . . And feel what it feels like . . . In your body . . . Feel what it feels like . . . In your mind . . . To know that you have already achieved what it is that you want to achieve, and are now living your life the way you want to live . . . Appreciating, and savoring any positive thoughts or feelings that are coming up for you in this moment . . . That's right . . .

*Then . . . When you are ready . . . You can allow a part of your mind to float up out of this moment . . . And float back in time . . . To that moment when you sat in meditation at the end of the MORE program . . . And then play the movie of your life forward from that point there . . . To this point here . . . Now that you have achieved what it is that you want to achieve, and are now living your life the way you want to live . . . You can see the steps that you began to take to get from that point there . . . To this point here . . . You can see yourself putting what you have learned into action . . . Successfully . . . You can see the positive changes you made, one step at a time . . . How you began to live your life more mindfully . . . Reappraising more . . . Facing challenges differently . . . Responding more effectively to stressors and pain . . . With inner strength and wisdom . . . And appreciating the good things in life . . . Savoring more . . . Living more meaningfully . . . Thriving . . . Empowered . . . To achieve what it is that you want to achieve, and live your life the way you want to live . . . That's right . . . And you can rewind . . . And review . . . And replay the best parts of this experience . . . Again and again . . . So you can learn what you need to learn . . . Now . . . [**Therapist note**: As the therapist now you should pause and be silent for 30–60 seconds.] That's right . . . And when you know how you can use what you've learned from this experience to help yourself, and help those that you love, in future moments . . . You will feel a little more comfortable, a little more centered, and a little more hopeful . . . When you complete this practice.*

Process the Future Pacing and Imagery Rehearsal (Using PURER)

What did you like best about that experience? Was there anything challenging about it?

Closing

You've grown so much over these past weeks. Through hard work and disciplined practice, you've strengthened your mindfulness. You've learned to reappraise the painful parts of life and savor life's beauty. You know how to find meaning in the face of life's challenges. This meaning will continue to fuel your recovery. This is just the beginning of your healing journey, not the end. I know you have what it takes to keep on growing, to live the kind of life you want to live. I believe in you!

Common Pitfalls, Troubleshooting, and Closing Advice for the Therapist

Helping patients to first develop a specific and actionable recovery plan, and then helping them to envision enacting this plan effectively, is the key to making this session successful. Patients need to have a clear sense of how they will apply skills they learned from the program to address their own personal triggers and risk factors. During the development of the mindful recovery plan, if patients are struggling to identify their own triggers, coping strategies, or reasons for recovery, you can foster group dialogue and seek input from others. The final technique in the session is a future pacing or age progression technique with a heavy hypnotic flavor (Erickson et al., 1976). While mindfulness is decidedly about focusing on the present, this final technique orients patients into the future, to envision themselves as empowered, thriving in recovery. This technique also involves the use of imagery for cognitive-behavioral skill rehearsal, guiding the patient to imagine using the mindfulness, reappraisal, and savoring skills they have learned in the program to help themselves in the future. Take your time to deliver each suggestion slowly, giving patients time to fully imagine and experience themselves in this empowered state.

It's important to have a plan of what to do when things get tough. Without a plan, stressors can start to pile up fast and the next thing you know, you may feel totally overwhelmed. It might seem like it's impossible to get your pain or opioid use under control again. But if you have a plan of how you can address challenges as they arise, when problems occur things won't completely fall apart. You can tackle them head on, and be proactive instead of reactive. There are five important steps to coming up with a mindful recovery plan:

1. Identifying triggers
2. Identifying strategies to address each trigger
3. Identifying a plan to continue your mindfulness practice
4. Identifying what you can do if you experience a lapse
5. Identifying your reasons for recovery

Section 1. Identifying Your Triggers

In the past, when you experienced bad pain flare-ups or significant increases in opioid use, what kinds of things were happening in your life at those times? What activating events, beliefs/thoughts, emotions, or people may have triggered you?

_____

_____

_____

_____

Section 2. Identifying Strategies to Address Each Trigger

How can you use what you have learned to manage triggers, stress, pain flare-ups, and the urge to take more opioids?

_____

_____

_____

_____

(cont.)

Section 3. Identifying a Plan to Continue Your Mindfulness Practice

How will you continue your regular practice of mindfulness, reappraisal, and savoring on your own? When will you practice? What days and times? How can you remind yourself to practice? How can you stay motivated to practice? Which people in your life can support you and encourage you to practice?

_____

_____

_____

_____

Section 4. Identifying What You Can Do If You Experience a Lapse

Instead of thinking, "Now that I've blown my progress, everything is over. I might as well just forget it, and go back to my old way of dealing with things," what would be a more helpful way of thinking about a lapse? If you do have a lapse, what steps can you take to resume your recovery plan?

_____

_____

_____

Section 5. Identifying Your Reasons for Recovery

What are your reasons for recovery? What motivated you to start this course, and to stick with it? Who are the important people in your life? What kind of a person do you really want to be? What are your values? What actions do you need to do, and what ideas do you need to hold on to to live a meaningful life and to live your life the way you want to live?

_____

_____

_____

Chapter 7

Supplemental Session
on Self-Transcendence in Recovery

> Once the island consisting of the idea of the body has been washed away, once
> singleness of thought has been attained in the pure river of consciousness, and
> when, on the other hand, you have retained the host of senses in your inner
> being, [then] do you appear, one, eternal, the essence of everything.
> —BHATTADIVĀKARAVATSA (cited in Bansat-Boudon & Tripathi, 2014, p. 216)

As discussed in Chapter 6, we have found there are therapists and MORE participants who become interested in extending the work they have been doing in practicing mindfulness. For those readers, this chapter describes an additional supplemental session that could be offered after Session 7 and before the final closing session on "Maintaining Mindful Recovery." In the MORE program, Session 7 introduces the concept of interdependence, the notion that all things depend on one another for their existence and therefore derive meaning and purpose from these relations. Developing a strong sense of our connections to the world at large, a strong sense that we are not independent and isolated "islands" in a sea of humanity, allows us to deepen the benefits of mindfulness practice, and presents opportunities to view our self as expansive, as much more than our experiences of pain and addiction. In Chapter 2 we discussed how the sense of self can become entangled with chronic pain and addiction. For instance, if one says, "I am in pain" enough times, the preposition *in* eventually gets dropped, and "I am in pain" becomes "I am pain" as the sense of self becomes identified with chronic pain. We become attached to and defined by a pain-laden identity. Similarly, we can come to feel defined and marked by addiction, as if the shame of addictive behavior has sullied our very nature. We come to mistakenly believe we are broken and flawed. But mindfulness can help us to let go of and transcend this form of attachment, allowing us to view ourselves as deeply interconnected with something greater than our limited sense of identity, something more fundamental. When we do this, we access our basic goodness. "Every human being has a basic nature of goodness, which is undiluted and unconfused. That goodness contains tremendous gentleness

> Mindfulness helps us
> transcend the view of the
> self as broken and flawed.

and appreciation . . . we have an actual connection to reality that can wake us up and make us feel basically, fundamentally good" (Trungpa, 1985, p. 31).

The MORE program has been designed to point to this basic goodness through the various mindfulness, reappraisal, and savoring techniques and PURER processing approach embedded in each session. But the arc of positive psychological states specified in the mindfulness-to-meaning theory (MMT) reaches its zenith in self-transcendence—the sense of being connected to something greater than the self—a fundamental ground of being that is the source of basic goodness. Thus, in this chapter, we expand beyond the idea of interdependence by directly investigating self-transcendence and why it is germane to, and even part of, the recovery process.

Leaders of the Western human potential movement that antedated modern mindfulness therapy and positive psychology, including Abraham Maslow, Fritz Perls, and Viktor Frankl, hinted at self-transcendence more than 70 years ago. Of course, psychological science stumbled upon this dimension centuries and millennia after masters of esoteric wisdom like Abhinavagupta, Chuang-Tzu, Garab Dorje, Kṣemaraāja, Meister Eckhart, Moses ben Jacob Cordovero, Namgyal, Rumi, and Adi Shankara put forth taxonomies and technologies of self-transcendence in the treatises of multiple mystical traditions. For convenient designation and ease of understanding, I use a common label of "self-transcendence" for the range of phenomena catalogued by these sages, though to be clear, self-transcendence may have many gradations and specific qualia, leading to various forms of expression in human experience. It is beyond the scope of the present volume to parse the phenomenology of these rarefied states, and indeed, masterworks of contemplative geniuses (e.g., Abhinavagupta, 1987) have done so far beyond the capabilities of Western science and psychotherapy. For our purposes, I simply note that MORE, as a therapeutic approach, focuses on restructuring reward processing from the valuation of drug reward back to the valuation of natural reward, and points toward self-transcendence as a potential path for healing and self-actualization.

These ancient contemplative traditions converge on a deceptively simple idea: When we transcend our limited sense of self, we taste the basic goodness of our one true nature. According to the Buddhist Mahāmudrā sage Gampopa, meditating on this one taste (*ekarāsa* in Sanskrit) leads to "understanding diverse appearances as being one, from the standpoint of their intrinsic nature" (Ray, 2002, p. 280). That intrinsic nature, in the Nondual Shaiva Tantra sutras of Kṣemaraāja, is *awareness*—a foundational principle that "brings about the fusion of everything in complete nonduality, causing one to relish all things as a seamless unity" (Wallis, 2017, p. 60). Dzogchen characterizes this fundamental phenomenological substrate as "the supreme source of everything, pure and total consciousness," "the self-arising wisdom," the "fundamental substance of all phenomena," "primordial self-perfection," and the "bliss of the authentic non-dual condition [that] contains all forms" (Norbu & Clemente, 1999, pp. 138–141). This blissfully aware substrate can be experienced, and "tasted," like all tastes, through the savoring that emerges from deep mindfulness practice. Unlike some psychological models and religions that view the human mind or soul as inherently broken and inevitably flawed (and thus in need of salvation or redemption by the Divine), this worldview holds that at its heart, our fundamental nature is undivided, pure, perfect, and free, a spacious plenum totally full and complete, a seamless unity with the whole of existence.

> Awareness savors itself during deep mindfulness practice.

This view stands in contrast with our normative experience as a self. We typically experience ourselves as isolated subjects, identified with our bodies and encapsulated by our skin, seeking out the objects of the world that we desire. "I" am inside here (located somewhere in the head) and the world is out there. But from the contemplative perspective articulated above, we are not separate and isolated from the world as limited and deficient selves who crave and seek out what we desire to fulfill our incomplete and broken natures. Instead, these wisdom traditions hold that the perceived separateness of an abiding, individual self, of the "skin encapsulated ego" (Watts, 1961/1989, p. 9), is an illusion generated by the intricacies of the human nervous system interacting with culture and language—that is, the duality of self and world is only epistemological, but not ontological. According to the Advaita Vedanta of Shankara, it is like when in dim light one mistakes a rope for a snake; we superimpose our concept of an individual self separate from the world upon a more fundamental unity (Deutsch & Dalvi, 2004).

In contrast, our true nature is indivisibly one with the whole of existence. According to systems theory, the individual and its environment are structurally coupled to each other through the transfer of biochemical energy across a membrane demarcating the boundaries of the organism, a membrane that is made of the very same material as its environment (Maturana & Varela, 1987); and thus, self and world are one continuous process, a unified field. Or as Alan Watts (1961/1989) articulated,

> My outline, which is not just the outline of my skin but of every organ and cell in my body, is also the inline of the world. The movements of this outline are my movements, but they are also movements of the world—of its inline. . . . Seeing this, I *feel with* the world. (p. 65)

This field connects all that exists, as described in the words of 13th-century Jewish mystic Moses de Leon, as a

> unified oneness . . . a chain linking everything from the highest to the lowest. . . . There is nothing—not even the tiniest thing—that is not fasted to the links of this chain. Everything is catenated in its mystery, caught in its oneness. . . . The entire chain is one. Down to the last link, everything is linked with everything else. (cited in Matt, 1995, p. 26)

However, our ignorance of this view causes suffering, in that through its obscuration, we see ourselves as lacking and flawed. The process of recognizing one's true nature has been likened to looking into a mirror that reflects the world (Abhinavagupta, 1987). This mirror reflects the world in a distorted way when it becomes dusty and clouded by ego and destructive emotions. But when the mirror is cleared through moments of deep meditation, the meditator transcends the limited sense of self and "sees the mass of existent things, beings, feelings, and mental states dissolving into the Sky of Awareness like wisps of autumn cloud" (Wallis, 2017, p. 395). The self-transcendent state reveals the surface of the mirror, and it becomes evident, as Abhinavagupta points out, that within awareness "this entire universe manifests like a variegated image inside a mirror. Consciousness, however, becomes aware of the universe by the activity of its own awareness" (Kaul, 2020, p. 168). Like a mirror in which the apparent multiplicity of separate objects and events are manifested in a single unitary reflection, awareness reveals the diversity of reality as a unity. But, unlike an object reflected in a mirror, the universe is constituted by the activity of awareness. So, the metaphor of a canvas on which the image of the universe is painted might perhaps be more apt, as expressed by Abhinavagupta's disciple Kṣemaraāja:

Awareness unfolds the universe on the canvas that is Herself. . . . She unfolds the universe as if it were separate and different from Herself, though in actuality, it is not separate, just like an image of a city reflected in a mirror [is not separate from the mirror]. Therefore it is taught here that the world exists in a state of oneness with the Light of Awareness. (Wallis, 2017, p. 73)

> The self-transcendent state reveals the surface of the mirror of awareness.

Outside of the realm of philosophy, modern psychological scientists have conceptualized two forms of self-transcendence: relational transcendence and annihilational transcendence (Yaden et al., 2017). In relational transcendence, one experiences the fundamental unity between self and world. During moments of intense attentional absorption, there is a sense of merging or mingling of subject and object into an oceanic boundlessness. Practically, such experiences can occur during the deep communion that arises during savoring aesthetic or meaningful life experiences.

On the other hand, annihilational self-transcendence involves the dissolution of the sense of self and emptying of the distinction between observer and observed. Another term used for this experience is *nondual awareness*—a term that provides some additional interpretation for the academically inclined. Nondual awareness involves a temporary experiential collapse of the subject–object dichotomy that organizes ordinary human consciousness. Awareness may be said to be "nondual" when the normal duality of subject and object that structures our waking experience is transcended. In moments of nondual awareness, the normal sense of self begins to fade. This dissolution of the ego is often followed by the phenomenology of an empty spaciousness, the sense that consciousness is nonlocalized and all pervasive, like the open space of the sky, and "the I-centeredness falls away, there is no longer a center or periphery to awareness." (Kabat-Zinn, 2005, p. 169). Of this phenomenon, the Mahāmudrā tradition provides the following descriptor: "Mind is similar to space. It has the nature of space. It is equivalent to space" (Namgyal, 2019, p. 233). Like space, a mind empty of the limited sense of self can contain all things.

Yet, this absence of independent self is not characterized by a nihilistic emptiness, bereft of life. To the contrary, self-transcendence and nondual awareness are marked by the qualia of a luminous cognizance full of affective bliss. This uniform mass of blissful consciousness, known as *cidānandaikaghana* in Nondual Shaiva Tantra (Bansat-Boudon & Tripathi, 2014), is experienced as limitless fullness, a sense of all-pervading love, grace, and connection that motivates compassion. Thus, at its zenith, the experience of self-transcendence carries the sense of ultimate meaningfulness and reward (Austin, 1999). And indeed, of this state it is spoken in the *Sivasutra*, "When the yogi is established in pure awareness, his craving is destroyed . . . thus he savors his own inherently blissful nature which illumines itself with the rays of its consciousness. . . . Thus [at] the very moment the yogi abandons the craving" (Dyczkowski, 1992, pp. 163–164). Given this latter point, it is unsurprising that MORE, as a therapeutic approach focused on restructuring reward processing from valuation of drug reward back to valuation of natural reward, would point toward transcendence as a potential path for healing and self-actualization.

We can experience brief tastes of self-transcendence when we are at a concert of our favorite band, and we become so fully absorbed, so lost in the music and the lights that we lose all sense of ourselves, and melt into the thrilling bliss of the musical notes. These experiences can occur in nature, such as when we are watching a gorgeous sunset at sea, feeling a deep sense of awe and interconnectedness to the world around us, when the sense of self becomes totally quiet and is eclipsed by a feeling of expansiveness and limitlessness. These experiences can occur under the influence of psychedelic compounds like psilocybin or LSD. And they can and do occur during meditation.

It was empirical data that indicated the need to evolve MORE to point directly toward self-transcendence. After hearing hundreds of anecdotal reports of patients in MORE therapy groups describing spontaneous self-transcendent experiences during the PURER process, in 2018 my colleagues and I published psychometric research to validate the use of a self-report measure to quantify experiences of self-transcendence called the Nondual Awareness Dimensional Assessment (Hanley et al., 2018). When validating this instrument, we began to collect data on self-transcendent experiences occasioned by MORE, and found, much to our surprise, that, consistent with their qualitative reports, patients in MORE reported significant increases in the intensity and frequency of self-transcendent experiences, including ego dissolution, unity, and bliss (Garland, Hanley, Riquino, et al., 2019; Garland, Hanley, Hudak, et al., 2022; Hudak et al., 2021). Even more critically, these increases in self-transcendence were statistically associated with decreased chronic pain severity (Garland, Hanley, Riquino, et al., 2019) and altered brain responses (i.e., enhanced frontal midline theta power) that led to reduced opioid use (Hudak et al., 2021) and opioid misuse (Garland, Hanley, Hudak, et al., 2022). Our findings suggesting that meditation-induced self-transcendence could improve health outcomes were parallel to other emerging data demonstrating that psychedelic drugs (e.g., psilocybin, ketamine) produce clinical benefits by eliciting self-transcendent experiences (Dakwar et al., 2018; Griffiths et al., 2016; Rothberg et al., 2021). Once discovering that self-transcendent experiences were linked with clinical improvement, it became evident to me that self-transcendence was an untapped therapeutic mechanism that could be leveraged and optimized by directly pointing to those states in the MORE program.

To be clear, self-transcendence is not an all-or-nothing phenomenon. Rather, self-transcendent experiences likely exist along a continuum, from experiencing the self as the skin-encapsulated ego (the absence of self-transcendence), to experiencing the self as more connected with others and the world (some self-transcendence), to experiencing an indivisible and seamless unity with all things (total self-transcendence) or a complete lack of subject–object duality (nonduality). Thus, meditation practitioners can achieve small tastes of self-transcendence (Austin, 1999), that, no matter how fleeting, may leave indelible marks on their future practice, serving as a beacon to light the way toward greater realization along the gradual path of meditation. Most patients do not experience total self-transcendence during the MORE meditation; such a complete mystical experience is quite rare. Nevertheless, even the taste of a mild self-transcendent state can be experienced as healing.

> Self-transcendence is not an all-or-nothing phenomenon.

Yet these states are not a *certain* outcome of meditation. Just because one has a momentary experience of transcending the limited sense of self or perceives their interconnectedness with the world during a given meditation practice session does not mean that one will experience these states the next time they meditate. In fact, these tastes of transcendence seem to occur spontaneously. They cannot be forced or intended but rather seem to arise under the right conditions (e.g., when one's meditation practice has been regular and disciplined). Chasing self-transcendence in meditation is not unlike trying to make yourself fall asleep: The harder you try, the more awake you become. But despite their transitory and elusive quality, even brief and partial tastes of self-transcendence may have important therapeutic value. They help us contact our basic goodness.

With respect to the treatment of chronic pain, opioid misuse, and addiction, self-transcendent experiences can be analgesic (Garland, Hanley, Riquino, et al., 2019; Hanley & Garland, 2022), and elicit brain signatures with anti-addictive properties (Garland, Hanley, Hudak, et al., 2022) that can help reduce opioid use (Hudak et al., 2021).

But where can one learn how best to stimulate tastes of self-transcendence? The canons of Mahāmudrā, Dzogchen, and Nondual Shaiva Tantra provide endless riches of knowledge in that regard. Drawing from many sources, in the supplemental session below is psychoeducational material and a meditation technique born out of my collaboration with my colleague Adam Hanley. These materials are intended to provide a means of "direct pointing" to self-transcendence. In the pointing-out instructions (ngo sprod) of Mahāmudrā (Namgyal, 2006) and Dzogchen (Rinpoche, 2013) traditions, the novitiate receives direct guidance in realizing the true nature of the mind as nondual awareness. This teaching approach accords with the "sudden school" of realization whereby the mind is assumed to possess the innate capacity to realize its nondual nature, in contrast to the more gradual, developmental path of renunciation and meditation held by many traditions to be necessary to achieve deep realization (Dunne, 2011). Thus, when the right instructions are given, realization of nondual awareness may be rapid, if not instantaneous, in certain sensitive individuals who are ready to receive the teaching. The session script that follows provides a hint. Admittedly, this is a fledgling attempt. From a scientific perspective, little is known about how to best facilitate the Western mind in attaining nondual awareness, and even less about how to help people suffering from addiction, distress, and chronic pain realize tastes of self-transcendence. We still have much to learn in terms of pointing toward self-transcendence, but I hope this material may be of benefit to the field as a means of alleviating suffering and evolving consciousness toward true and abiding flourishing.

> Self-transcendent states can help heal pain and opioid use.

Agenda

Mindfulness-of-pain practice: 20 minutes

Process in-session mindfulness-of-pain practice (using PURER): 5 minutes

Process mindfulness home practice and STOP (using PURER): 5 minutes

Process reappraisal home practice (using PURER): 5 minutes

Process savoring home practice (using PURER): 5 minutes

Break: 10 minutes

Tasting basic goodness through transcendence: 30 minutes

Mindfulness with direct pointing to transcendence: 25 minutes

Process mindfulness with direct pointing to transcendence (using PURER): 12 minutes

Assignment: 3 minutes—discuss and assign for the following week:

- Daily mindfulness of pain or body scan
- Daily reappraisal
- Daily savoring
- STOP

Materials Needed

A chime or bell (meditation bells or singing bowls work well)

Session Introduction for the Therapist

This material should be considered preliminary and under evolution. We have pilot-tested portions of this material in patients with chronic pain and those with full OUD in addiction recovery, and have found the material to be well received. We have also used portions of this material in preparatory and integration sessions for patients undergoing MORE combined with psychedelic-assisted therapy, to provide an experiential and conceptual map to guide patients through the self-transcendent states of consciousness that arise during the psychedelic experience. Keep in mind that this material is abstract and may be difficult for many patients to understand fully. The material provided is like the proverbial "finger pointing at the moon" from Zen Buddhism: It points the way to one's true nature, but each person must experience that truth in their own way, to the extent to which they are able to receive it, and at the right moment in their life. Such a realization cannot be forced, only suggested.

Session Script

Begin the session with the standard *mindfulness-of-pain* practice. Use the practice on pages 100–101 in Session 2.

Process the Mindfulness-of-Pain Practice (Using PURER)

What did you like best about that experience? Was there anything challenging about it?

Process the Mindfulness Home Practice (Using PURER)

How did you use mindfulness this week to help yourself with pain, opioid use (or addiction recovery)?

Process the STOP Practice

When you were focused on your breathing, what did you notice about your attention for the medication/drug? Did it keep getting pulled back to the medication/drug? What did you notice in your body when your attention was focused on the medication/drug? What thoughts did you notice? What did you do when you noticed your attention was captured by the medication/drug? Did you notice that you could bring your attention back to your breath, and keep it there longer? Did you find that you were more disinterested in the medication/drug, like you didn't care as much about it? Were you able to "step back" or practice "zooming out" during this experience? And were you able to use mindfulness, reappraisal, and savoring skills to manage pain and difficult feelings instead of relying on opioids?

Process the Reappraisal Home Practice

How did you use reappraisal this week to help yourself with stress, opioid use (or addiction recovery)?

Process the Savoring Home Practice

How did you use savoring this week to help yourself feel better or appreciate life more?

Tasting Basic Goodness through Transcendence

In Session 7 we asked you to zoom in to a raisin as a way to understand interdependence. If you zoomed in deeply enough, perhaps you could see the entire universe in a single raisin: the plant on which it grew, the rain that quenched its thirst, the rich dirt that provided it with nutrients, the insects and animals that fertilized that soil, the hands that picked the grape, and the sun and stars from which all of this matter and energy were born. If we look closely with mindfulness, we can see the universe contained within a single raisin. When we look closely with mindfulness, we can see that a raisin is not a separate, isolated, independent thing, but rather exists as a part of an interdependent network of relationships with all of the things that work together to produce it. The raisin exists only because of the soil, the rain, and the sun. So is the raisin separate and independent from these things? Or is it not?

On an even deeper level, on the level of atoms, a raisin is mostly empty space. Did you know that? Physics tells us that all objects are made of atoms. And atoms are tiny! Did you know that there are 10 million trillion atoms in a single grain of sand? But each atom is in turn made up of subatomic particles that are so tiny, that they take up only 0.01% of the volume of the atom. In other words, 99.99% of an atom is empty space. Because these tiny particles whirl around the atom so quickly, and because all of the atoms in an object are connected with one another through bonds of energy, it makes an object feel solid. But even the particles in an atom are not actually solid—they are made up of vibrations of energy. So if you could zoom in all the way, you would see that solid objects, like the raisin, are actually empty space filled with vibrating energy! And this energy fills all of space, almost like an ocean, and the objects we encounter around us are like waves on this ocean. They seem like separate things, but they are really all made of one thing: energy.

So zooming in all the way, we see that things are made of empty space filled with energy. Zooming out all the way, we see that what we call a "thing" is a net of relationships, connected to everything else. From this perspective, you could think of the entire universe like an ocean, with the waves being the individual things we perceive in the world, arising from and made up of the same basic energy of life.

Think about a forest. Have you ever walked in the forest and looked closely at the way trees grow from the ground? Trees grow up out of the rocks and soil. In a healthy forest, moss covers the bark of the tree and the rocks and the soil itself. When we look closely, we don't see a tree as separate from the moss as separate from the rock as separate from the soil. We see all of these things at once, all together. Take one away, and the tree would no longer live. If a tree was just floating in the vacuum of space, with no moss, rocks, and soil, would it live? No, of course not. Furthermore, the tree could not live without sunlight, without the carbon dioxide in the air, or without the rain that nourishes its roots. So we have this word *tree*, as if it were a separate, independent thing, but the tree would not exist without the net of interdependent relationships that we call "a forest." On the other hand, there would be no forests without trees. So trees and the forest are one thing, with two different names.

Of course, one could argue, why stop there? The rain comes from clouds, and clouds receive moisture from the ocean. The soil comes from the earth, and the matter from the earth was born in the heart of a star. So is a tree in the forest only a tree, or is the tree also the forest? Is a forest only a forest, or is a forest also a cloud and a star? The names we use divide these things up, but if they were really divided and separate, they could not live, they could not exist.

And what about you who observes the tree in the forest? Are you separate from the forest? You see the trees and moss and rocks and soil. But did you know that your vision is produced by light waves activating in nerve cells in the back of your brain? Without those cells, sight wouldn't be possible. And the same with sound, touch, smell, and taste—your senses arise from the activity of nerve cells in your brain interacting with some kind of vibration of energy in the world. You think you see a tree. But when you look out on the world, what you really see is the activity of the neurons in your brain interacting with vibrations of energy. And the cells of your brain are made up of matter, of atoms, that ultimately came from stars and space dust, just like the trees in the forest. So are you really separate from those things? Or are you the eyes of the world?

We usually think of ourselves as separate from the world, encased in our bodies, encapsulated by our skin. We think our self is somewhere behind the eyes, somewhere in the head. However, when you look out on the world, you can't see your head. It's like an invisible space. Instead of seeing your head, you see the world before you. But just like the tree in the forest, and just like the raisin in Session 7, you are connected to this world, to this vast net of energy and interdependence we call the universe. But, it can be easy to lose sight of your connection to everything, especially when experiences of pain or addiction leave you feeling hopelessly isolated and alone, giving you tunnel vision. But are you truly alone? Did you really come into this world isolated and alone?

As a wise philosopher once said, "We do not 'come into' this world; we come out of it, as leaves from a tree. As the ocean 'waves,' the Universe 'peoples.' Every individual is an expression of the whole realm of nature, a unique action of the total Universe" (Watts, 1959/2011, pp. 8–9). Think about waves on an ocean. You can watch an individual wave grow and move and crest on the surface of the sea. Each wave is an individual: Some waves are bigger, some waves are smaller, but all are made of the same stuff—water. The ocean is also made of water. So is the wave separate from the ocean? Is the ocean separate from the wave? No, of course not. The wave is the action of the ocean. In the same way, you are the activity of the universe perceiving itself.

Coming back to the idea of a tree in the forest, what about the bird that sings in the branches of the tree? When you hear the birdsong, are you really separate from the sound? Try listening to this sound now, with full mindfulness. [**Therapist note**: Play a chime or bell, or whistle or hum.] Is there a sound, and a separate self that hears the sound? Or is there just one thing, one experience, that we call hearing? Try again. [**Therapist note**: Play a chime or bell, or whistle or hum again.]

I started this discussion by describing discoveries about atoms and energy from powerful scientific instruments like electron microscopes. We typically think these scientific tools can help us to objectively see the world out there. But if you really think about it, everything that you see, hear, feel, and understand—you see, hear, feel, and understand those things through your mind. Every perception that you have, whether it's a sound in your ears, a feeling in your body, a sight through your eyes, or an image in a microscope or a telescope, you perceive it with your mind. The whole world "out there," and even your experience of your body, is really just a perception inside the mind. You can't ever step outside of that. So is the outside of the world outside, or inside? Is the inside of the mind inside, or outside?

It's like watching a movie on a movie screen. You see people, objects, buildings, the landscape, the sky, the clouds, and the sun, but all of those things are just images on a screen. All of those images are made of one substance: They are made of light. They appear to be separate objects moving on the screen, but in reality, the image is one thing: light projected on a screen. And the screen exists independent of the images. We don't usually notice the screen because we are so captivated by the images. We become focused on the faces we see, of people crying, screaming, or laughing. We get caught up in the drama of the story.

In this way, the mind is like a screen, canvas, or a mirror that contains the image of the world. Like a mirror, the mind reflects everything in your experience. You could not experience the world without the mind. All that you see, the world you experience, is reflected in your mind, just as objects are reflected in a mirror. The true, original nature of the mind, like a mirror, is perfectly clear, totally open, receiving all that comes before it. Totally pure, with the quality of basic goodness. But over time, the mirror of the mind can become dirty. Our painful life experiences and traumas, our habits, and our cravings begin to cloud the mind as dust and grime can cloud the surface of a mirror. After years, and decades, we can no longer see clearly but instead only see a distorted reflection, biased by negative beliefs rooted in the sense that we are flawed human beings. As we come to identify with pain and addiction more and more, these forms of suffering become the central theme of our life story. This process of identification clouds the mind's mirror and prevents us from seeing our true self. But the mirror can be cleaned. Mindfulness can allow us to clear the mirror of the mind, and to look directly into its untarnished surface.

When we look at the surface of the mirror, we see that its true nature, beneath the dirt and grime, and beneath the images being reflected, is open, clear, spotless, stainless, pure, and free. It reflects all things. In this way, the true nature of the mind is totally open, like space, able to hold and contain all things. This is the part of you that's always been there, despite all of the changes and challenges of your life. It's the part of you that's observing all the parts of your life, the observing awareness.

Reflect back on that awareness, as if you were looking in to a mirror. You might think of the observing awareness as that mirror that reflects the image of your life. And of course you would not know life without awareness. Awareness is what allows you to experience everything. So it is true to say that all experiences occur within the field of awareness. And therefore, awareness is your true nature, your true self. So everything that happens, happens in awareness, and in this way, everything is a part of you, just as you are a part of everything. In this sense then, awareness is the energy of life. All the changes, all the activity, all the events that you've experienced in your life, you've experienced through awareness. So, there is this part of you that is bigger than any one experience. There's a part of you that is beyond pain and addiction. It's the deep part of you, the observing awareness, that contains all experience but is not defined or marked by them. It's the open, reflective, spotless, stainless space of awareness that we've talked about before, like the space of the sky, the spaces in between thoughts and feelings. That's the part of the mirror that is wiped clean during meditation, that's free and full of possibility.

As you may have experienced during previous mindfulness practice sessions, there are moments when you are able to let go of your sense of self. Where the ideas you had about yourself, the stories that you told yourself about who you are, start to quiet down, or even fade away completely. In these moments, we can go beyond our self. This is the moment of self-transcendence, of connecting with something greater than your self. Perhaps you have caught glimpses of that during your mindfulness sessions. Perhaps the feeling that your self extends far beyond your body, into the world, into the universe, or beyond. Maybe the feeling that you are deeply connected with everything that surrounds you, perhaps connected to all things. Perhaps a sense of your mind as being totally open, totally clear, like space, like an empty mirror. The mirror reflects the clear light of life, the light of the sun, shining. Awareness filled with peace, filled with light, filled with the energy of life. Your basic goodness. In these moments, we are totally complete, we need nothing, we are completely fulfilled. These moments reveal our true nature, our true self, and the meaning of our life.

Of course, we cannot stay in these moments forever. In fact, the harder we try to make them happen, or hold on to them, the more quickly they slip away. We can't make them last forever, but they can have lasting impact on us. When we have a moment of self-transcendence, that moment can help us to reflect and decide who we want to be, to rewrite our life story. Think of the moment of self-transcendence as a moment of wiping the mirror clean. A chance to see your basic goodness shining within. You can get a fresh start, in any moment, and write the next chapter of your life.

We end today's session with a practice that uses some of the same zooming-in and zooming-out techniques we've been practicing, but instead of examining pain or craving, we will practice mindfulness of the self, and of self-transcendence. We will hold up the mirror.

Mindfulness with Direct Pointing to Transcendence

Sitting comfortably but regally, as if you are a king or queen, with your spine straight and belly relaxed, you can allow your eyes to close . . . or they can remain open and relaxed on a spot in front of you. You can begin to notice the sensation of the body resting in the chair . . . of the legs and back making contact with the cushion of the chair . . . And we have this word contact, but what is it really? . . . A sensation of warmth? Or heaviness? Or tingling? Can you really tell where your body ends, and the world begins? . . . Or where the world ends, and your body begins? . . . Do you feel the world? . . . Do you feel your body? . . . Are these two different sensations, or one? . . . Is there a separation between yourself and the world? . . . Or is there just one experience?

And when you are ready, shifting the focus of the attention to the breath . . . Noticing the natural sensation of the breath . . . Moving into the nostrils . . . Just noticing the temperature of that air . . . It's warmth or coolness . . . or perhaps becoming aware of the movement of the breath deeper in the body, filling the lungs . . . That's right . . . Becoming aware of the beginning of each breath . . . Becoming aware of the ending of each breath . . . And the space between . . . From which the breaths arise . . . And to which they return, all on their own . . . Is there a separation between the breath and that space? . . . Where does the breath stop, and the space begin? . . . And if the mind begins to wander . . . to thoughts or feelings . . . Becoming aware that they too have a beginning . . . And an ending . . . Becoming aware of the space from which the thoughts and feelings arise . . . And to which they return, all on their own . . . Is there a separation between your thoughts and that space? . . . Where does the space stop and the thought begin? . . . Is there a separation between your feelings and that space? . . . And where does the space stop and the feeling begin? . . .

Becoming aware of the space within the body. . . . Is there a separation between the body and that inner space? . . . Then becoming aware of the space outside the body . . . The space around the body . . . Enveloping the body . . . That's right . . . Is there a separation between the body and that outer space? . . . And then, wondering, is the space inside the body, and the space outside the body, two different spaces, or one? Is there a limit to this space? . . . Does it have a center? . . . Does it have edges? Are there spaces inside that space where the space is not? Resting the body in that space, now . . .

Becoming aware of the space within awareness . . . . That's right . . . Is there a separation between awareness and that inner space? . . . Can you become aware of space outside awareness? . . . Is there a separation between awareness and that outer space? . . . Is there a limit to awareness? . . . Does awareness have a center? . . . Does it have edges? . . . Are there spaces inside awareness where awareness is not? And is the space inside awareness, and the space outside awareness, two different spaces, or one? And is awareness space? . . . Or space awareness? . . . Is it not? Resting awareness in that space, now . . . The open space of mindfulness . . .

Does this space of awareness have a shape? . . . A form? . . . A color? . . . Is it fixed? . . . Or changing? . . . Does it have a location or direction? . . . Is it supported by, or resting upon, something external? . . . Is it supported by, or resting upon, something internal? . . . Can it be pointed to at all? . . . Is this space of awareness empty? . . . Or full? . . . Or both? . . . Is this space of awareness clear? . . . Is it clear like light radiating from the sun or moon? . . . Or is it clear without a color or light? . . . Clear like an empty mirror? . . .

And soon you may begin to notice that thoughts and feelings are like clouds passing in this space, the space of a clear blue sky . . . Like clouds drifting, thoughts, and feelings, and sensations come out of nowhere, gradually change shape, and then fade into the distance . . . And there is no need to hold on to those thoughts or push them away . . . They just vanish into space . . . Like clouds . . . They go nowhere and reside nowhere . . . All that appears in the mind . . . are only appearances . . . Radiating from the mind . . . like light from the sun . . . And a part of the mind is like those thoughts passing like clouds . . . But there is a deeper part of the mind . . . that is more like . . . the space in which the clouds pass . . . the space filled with the light of the sun . . . the space of observing awareness . . . that is open . . . boundless . . . luminous . . . and free . . . just watching, just observing . . . peacefully . . . Always here . . . Inside of every moment . . . Underneath everything . . . Inside of everything . . . Surrounding everything . . . One with everything . . . And you can focus your attention on that part of your mind, or you can continue to focus your attention on your breathing . . . That's right . . . And now, you can take a few long moments to focus on any positive experiences that have come up during this practice . . . Feelings of warmth . . . or tingling . . . or vibration . . . A blissful mass of consciousness . . . Your basic goodness . . . The energy of life . . . Like the heart of the sun . . . An uninterrupted flow, like a river . . . Yet stable like a mountain . . . pulsating . . . expanding . . . Appreciating and savoring whatever positive feelings have arisen during this practice . . . or continuing to focus on the breath . . . That's right . . . And when you know that each time that you practice this . . . It will become easier and easier to go even more deeply into the state of mindfulness . . . Then you may feel a little more centered, a little more comfortable, and a little more complete . . . when you open your eyes and return your attention to the room.

Process Mindfulness with Direct Pointing to Transcendence (Using PURER)

What did you like best about that experience? Was there anything challenging about it? When I asked whether you could sense the separation between yourself and the chair, what did you notice? When I asked you to imagine that the space inside your body and the space outside your body were one space, what happened next? When I pointed out that thoughts and feelings come and go within the space of awareness, and that the space is always there, one with everything, what did you experience? When I invited you to notice blissful feelings, what did you sense? What does this experience tell you about your true self? What does this experience have to do with recovery?

Home Practice

- Daily mindfulness-of-pain or body scan practice
- Daily reappraisal practice (with Handout S3.2)
- Daily savoring practice
- STOP

Conclusion

This final chapter discussed self-transcendence as a new frontier in the treatment of chronic pain and addiction. Yet, self-transcendence—the experience of connectedness to something greater than the self—has been classically construed as the *sine qua non* of addiction recovery (e.g., surrendering to a higher power in Alcoholics Anonymous [AA]). This notion makes sense through the lens of neuroscience. During meditative self-transcendent experiences, the default mode network appears to become more connected with the dorsal attentional and salience networks in the brain—reducing the normative anticorrelation between extrinsic (i.e., brain regions devoted to processing sensory information from the external world "out there") and intrinsic (i.e., brain regions involved in processing self-referential thought and the internal world "in our heads"; Froeliger et al., 2012; Josipovic, 2014) networks. Representations of self and the world become more integrated in the brain, and thus, from a neurobiological perspective we become connected to something greater than the self. These patterns of brain connectivity are not unlike those observed during the experience of ego dissolution induced by psychedelic drugs (Tagliazucchi et al., 2016). In this way, self-transcendence may induce self-referential plasticity, opening the self to novel sets of information from which a new autobiographical narrative can be authored, a life story that is marked by the sense of meaning and resilience in the face of adversity. In view of the role of aberrant self-referential processing in chronic pain and addiction, modulating functional connectivity patterns via mindfulness-induced self-transcendent experiences might "reset" default mode network dysfunction, freeing the individual from maladaptive cognitive-affective habits and opening a path toward personal transformation and psychological growth.

Yet, ultimately this healing process is not limited to habit patterns in the brain. The very notion of self-transcendence points to the idea that who we truly are, our true nature, is not dictated by our past conditioning. Indeed, the self-transcendent state has been labeled "unconditioned" (Namgyal, 2006). To the extent that chronic pain and addiction arise out of a history of dysfunctional patterns of learning in the brain, the experience of self-transcendence may provide a means of freedom from our conditioned responses. Thus, throughout the MORE program we have characterized the "observing awareness" as "open," "clear," "spotless," "stainless," and "free." The experience of freedom, no matter how fleeting, may help to counter the gyre of the downward spiral and stimulate an upward spiral of positive cognition and affect toward eudaimonic well-being and flourishing in life (Garland, Fredrickson, et al., 2010).

Insofar as self-transcendence marks the apex of the mindfulness-to-meaning theory (MMT), we have come to a natural conclusion in our discussion of MORE as a treatment for chronic pain, opioid misuse, and addiction. Of course, this book represents a beginning, not an end, to learning about how mindfulness, reappraisal, and savoring may be used to enhance the recovery process (see the Appendix for additional resources for learning about the philosophy, science, and practices underlying MORE). In the same way that you would encourage your patients to practice the mind–body skills in MORE to strengthen their recovery, I encourage you to practice your skills in delivering the MORE program to strengthen your ability to implement this evidence-based treatment with fidelity and competence. In time, you will internalize the structure and the processing approach, as well as the philosophy and ethos of the MORE intervention, and make this material your own. May we hold up the mirror, and never forget our higher purpose on this path, remembering the truth about why we are doing this life-saving work in the service of compassion. We too are part of the whole.

Appendix

Resources for Learning MORE

This book represents the beginning of your journey as a MORE therapist, not the end. There are many resources for you to learn more about MORE, mindfulness, and therapy for chronic pain, opioid misuse, and OUD. I have highlighted a number of those resources here. In addition, I encourage you to refer to the reference section of this book that will lead you to many additional sources where you can both educate yourself, as well as your patients, about the process of recovery and healing.

Training and Certification

First and foremost, I strongly encourage you to receive formal training in MORE. Although reading and following this book will prepare you to deliver MORE in your practice, participating in training will allow you to hone your MORE facilitation skills and significantly increase your competence as a MORE therapist. Although MORE is a manualized therapy, the PURER approach cannot be manualized, and training will help model the most effective use of PURER in clinical practice. Training will also greatly refine your ability to deliver the mind–body techniques in MORE. As of April 2024, I am the only person offering training in MORE (although this will change over the next several years as other MORE therapists achieve the credentialing needed to become a trainer). To date, I have trained more than 900 clinicians from around the United States and internationally. Training information can be found at *https://drericgarland.com/training-in-more*.

I hold several trainings online each year. In addition, health care organizations and agencies (including your own) can contact me to organize an agency-specific training at your location. Participants receive intensive didactic and experiential instruction in implementing the mindfulness, reappraisal, and savoring skills integral to MORE. Participants practice the therapeutic techniques outlined in this book via clinical role plays, and receive live supervision in the delivery of therapeutic techniques via real-time feedback to optimize the delivery of the MORE intervention.

Certification in MORE requires completion of basic and advanced trainings, as well as demonstration of fidelity to the model (i.e., adequate levels of therapist competence and adherence to the protocol on the MORE Fidelity Measure; Hanley & Garland, 2021).

Mindfulness

I recommend these writings to gain a stronger understanding of the Western conceptualization of mindfulness and the science of mindfulness. These classic pieces will give you an entry point into understanding the concept from a Western psychological perspective:

Brown, K. W., Creswell, J. D., & Ryan, R. M. (Eds.). (2015). *Handbook of mindfulness: Theory, research, and practice.* Guilford Press.

Kabat-Zinn, J. (1990). *Full catastrophe living.* Delacorte Press.

Kabat-Zinn, J. (2023). *Wherever you go, there you are: Mindfulness meditation in everyday life.* Hachette U.K.

Lutz, A., Slagter, H. A., Dunne, J. D., & Davidson, R. J. (2008). Attention regulation and monitoring in meditation. *Trends in Cognitive Sciences, 12,* 163–169.

Segal, Z., Williams, M., & Teasdale, J. (2013). *Mindfulness-based cognitive therapy for depression* (2nd ed.). Guilford Press.

Tang, Y.-Y., Hölzel, B. K., & Posner, M. I. (2015). The neuroscience of mindfulness meditation. *Nature Reviews Neuroscience, 16*(4), 213–225.

Vago, D. R., & Silbersweig, D. A. (2012). Self-awareness, self-regulation, and self-transcendence (S-ART): A framework for understanding the neurobiological mechanisms of mindfulness. *Frontiers in Human Neuroscience, 6,* 296.

Zeidan, F., Martucci, K. T., Kraft, R. A., Gordon, N. S., McHaffie, J. G., & Coghill, R. C. (2011). Brain mechanisms supporting the modulation of pain by mindfulness meditation. *Journal of Neuroscience, 31*(14), 5540–5548.

Conceptual and Philosophical Foundations

I recommend these texts to strengthen your understanding of the philosophical approaches, psychological models, and neuroscience frameworks that informed the development of MORE:

Aurelius, M. (2015). *Meditations.* Penguin.

Bansat-Boudon, L., & Tripathi, K. D. (2014). *An introduction to Tantric philosophy: The Paramârthasâra of Abhinavagupta with the commentary of Yogarâja.* Routledge.

Bateson, G. (1972). *Steps to an ecology of mind.* University of Chicago Press.

Bryant, F. B., & Veroff, J. (2017). *Savoring: A new model of positive experience.* Psychology Press.

Donden, Y. (2022). *The Gospel of Garab Dorje: The highest, secret teachings of Tibetan Buddhism.* Lotus Press.

Dyczkowski, M. S. (1987). *The doctrine of vibration: An analysis of the doctrines and practices associated with Kashmir Shaivism.* SUNY Press.

Dyczkowski, M. S. (1992). *The aphorisms of Siva: The Siva Sutra with Bhaskara's commentary, the Varttika.* SUNY Press.

Erickson, M. H., Rossi, E. L., & Rossi, S. (1976). *Hypnotic realities.* Irvington.

Frankl, V. E. (1959). *Man's search for meaning.* Simon & Schuster. (Original work published 1946)

Hanh, T. N. (1988). *The sun my heart.* Parallax Press.

Keeney, B. P. (1983). *Aesthetics of change.* Guilford Press.

Koob, G. F., & Le Moal, M. (2001). Drug addiction, dysregulation of reward, and allostasis. *Neuropsychopharmacology, 24*(2), 97–129.

Laozi, & English, J. (2011). *Tao te ching.* Vintage.

Lazarus, R., & Folkman, S. (1984). *Stress, appraisal, and coping.* Springer.

Matt, D. C. (1995). *The essential Kabbalah: The heart of Jewish mysticism.* HarperCollins.

Maturana, H. R., & Varela, F. J. (1987). *The tree of knowledge: The biological roots of human understanding.* New Science Library/Shambhala.

Namgyal, D. T. (2006). *Mahamudra: The moonlight–quintessence of mind and meditation*. Simon & Schuster.

Norbu, C. N., & Clemente, A. (1999). *The supreme Source: The fundamental tantra of Dzogchen Semde Kunjed Gyalpo*. Shambhala.

Tiffany, S. T. (1990). A cognitive model of drug urges and drug-use behavior: Role of automatic and nonautomatic processes. *Psychological Review, 97*, 147–168.

Varela, F., Thompson, E., & Rosch, E. (1991). *The embodied mind: Cognitive science and human experience*. MIT Press.

Wallis, C. D. (2017). *The recognition sutras: Illuminating a 1,000-year-old spiritual masterpiece*. Mattamayura Press.

Watts, A. (1989). *Psychotherapy east and west*. New World Library. (Original work published 1961)

Watts, A. W. (2011). *The book: On the taboo against knowing who you are*. Vintage. (Original work published 1959)

Updates on MORE Research Program

For updates on the MORE research program, please visit my website, and in particular, the news page: *https://drericgarland.com/posts-news*. I blog about major MORE research findings and projects on this page to keep MORE therapists up-to-date.

References

Abhinavagupta. (1987). *Tantraloka: With the commentary of Jayaratha*. Motilal Banarsidass.

Agnoli, A., Xing, G., Tancredi, D. J., Magnan, E., Jerant, A., & Fenton, J. J. (2021). Association of dose tapering with overdose or mental health crisis among patients prescribed long-term opioids. *JAMA, 326*(5), 411–419.

Alshelh, Z., Marciszewski, K. K., Akhter, R., Di Pietro, F., Mills, E. P., Vickers, E. R., Peck, C. C., Murray, G. M., & Henderson, L. A. (2018). Disruption of default mode network dynamics in acute and chronic pain states. *NeuroImage: Clinical, 17,* 222–231.

American Psychiatric Association. (2013). *Diagnostic and statistical manual of mental disorders* (5th ed.). Author.

Anthony, W. A. (1993). Recovery from mental illness: The guiding vision of the mental health service system in the 1990s. *Psychosocial Rehabilitation Journal, 16*(4), 11–23.

Apkarian, A. V., Bushnell, M. C., Treede, R.-D., & Zubieta, J. K. (2005). Human brain mechanisms of pain perception and regulation in health and disease. *European Journal of Pain, 9*(4), 463–484.

Arch, J. J., Brown, K. W., Goodman, R. J., Della Porta, M. D., Kiken, L. G., & Tillman, S. (2016). Enjoying food without caloric cost: The impact of brief mindfulness on laboratory eating outcomes. *Behaviour Research and Therapy, 79,* 23–34.

Armentrout, D. P. (1979). The impact of chronic pain on the self-concept. *Journal of Clinical Psychology, 35*(3), 517–521.

Arnsten, A. F. T. (2009). Stress signalling pathways that impair prefrontal cortex structure and function. *Nature Reviews Neuroscience, 10*(6), 410–422.

Arvidsson, U., Dado, R. J., Riedl, M., Lee, J. H., Law, P. Y., Loh, H. H., Elde, R., & Wessendorf, M. W. (1995). Delta-opioid receptor immunoreactivity: Distribution in brainstem and spinal cord, and relationship to biogenic amines and enkephalin. *Journal of Neuroscience, 15*(2), 1215–1235.

Austin, J. H. (1999). *Zen and the brain: Toward an understanding of meditation and consciousness.* MIT Press.

Baer, R. A., Smith, G. T., Hopkins, J., Krietemeyer, J., & Toney, L. (2006). Using self-report assessment methods to explore facets of mindfulness. *Assessment, 13,* 27–45.

Baker, A. K., & Garland, E. L. (2019). Autonomic and affective mediators of the relationship between mindfulness and opioid craving among chronic pain patients. *Experimental and Clinical Psychopharmacology, 27*(1), 55–63.

Baldacchino, A., Balfour, D. J. K., Passetti, F., Humphris, G., & Matthews, K. (2012). Neuropsychological consequences of chronic opioid use: A quantitative review and meta-analysis. *Neuroscience and Biobehavioral Reviews, 36*(9), 2056–2068.

Baliki, M. N., Geha, P. Y., Apkarian, A. V., & Chialvo, D. R. (2008). Beyond feeling: Chronic pain hurts the brain, disrupting the default-mode network dynamics. *Journal of Neuroscience, 28*(6), 1398–1403.

Baliki, M. N., Mansour, A. R., Baria, A. T., & Apkarian, A. V. (2014). Functional reorganization of the default mode network across chronic pain conditions. *PLOS ONE, 9*(9), e106133.

Ballantyne, J. C., & Sullivan, M. D. (2017). Discovery of endogenous opioid systems: what it has meant for the clinician's understanding of pain and its treatment. *Pain, 158*(12), 2290–2300.

Baminiwatta, A., & Solangaarachchi, I. (2021). Trends and developments in mindfulness research over 55 years: A bibliometric analysis of publications indexed in Web of Science. *Mindfulness, 12,* 2099–2116.

Banich, M. T., & Caccamise, D. (2011). *Generalization of knowledge: Multidisciplinary perspectives.* Psychology Press.

Bansat-Boudon, L., & Tripathi, K. D. (2014). *An introduction to Tantric philosophy: The Paramârthasâra of Abhinavagupta with the commentary of Yogarâja.* Routledge.

Basbaum, A. I., & Fields, H. L. (1984). Endogenous pain control systems: Brainstem spinal pathways and endorphin circuitry. *Annual Review of Neuroscience, 7*(1), 309–338.

Bateson, G. (1971). The cybernetics of "self": A theory of alcoholism. *Psychiatry, 34*(1), 1–18.

Bateson, G. (1972). *Steps to an ecology of mind: Collected essays in anthropology, psychiatry, evolution, and epistemology.* University of Chicago Press.

Becerra, L., Harter, K., Gonzalez, R. G., & Borsook, D. (2006). Functional magnetic resonance imaging measures of the effects of morphine on central nervous system circuitry in opioid-naive healthy volunteers. *Anesthesia and Analgesia, 103*(1), 208–216.

Beck, A. T., Rush, A. J., Shaw, B. F., & Emery, G. (1979). *Cognitive therapy of depression.* Guilford Press.

Becker, W. C., & Fiellin, D. A. (2020). When epidemics collide: Coronavirus disease 2019 (COVID-19) and the opioid crisis. *Annals of Internal Medicine, 173*(1), 59–60.

Berridge, K. C., & Robinson, T. E. (2016). Liking, wanting, and the incentive-sensitization theory of addiction. *American Psychologist, 71*(8), 670–679.

Berridge, K. C., Robinson, T. E., & Aldridge, J. W. (2009). Dissecting components of reward: "Liking," "wanting," and learning. *Current Opinion in Pharmacology, 9,* 65–73.

Berryman, C., Stanton, T. R., Bowering, K. J., Tabor, A., McFarlane, A., & Moseley, G. L. (2014). Do people with chronic pain have impaired executive function? A meta-analytical review. *Clinical Psychology Review, 34*(7), 563–579.

Besson, J. M. (1999). The neurobiology of pain. *Lancet, 353*(9164), 1610–1615.

Bishop, G. H., & Landau, W. M. (1958). Evidence for a double peripheral pathway for pain. *Science, 128*(3326), 712–713.

Bishop, S. R., Lau, M., Shapiro, S., Carlson, L., Anderson, N. D., Carmody, J., Segal, Z. V., Abbey, S., Speca, M., Velting, D., & Devins, G. (2004). Mindfulness: A proposed operational definition. *Clinical Psychology: Science and Practice, 11,* 230–241.

Black, D. S., Christodoulou, G., & Cole, S. (2019). Mindfulness meditation and gene expression: A hypothesis-generating framework. *Current Opinion in Psychology, 28,* 302–306.

Bogaerts, K., Janssens, T., De Peuter, S., Van Diest, I., & Van den Bergh, O. (2009). Negative affective pictures can elicit physical symptoms in high habitual symptom reporters. *Psychology and Health, 25*(6), 685–698.

Bommersbach, T., Ross, D. A., & Aquino, J. P. D. (2020). Perpetual hunger: The neurobiological consequences of long-term opioid use. *Biological Psychiatry, 87*(1), e1–e3.

Borsook, D., Youssef, A. M., Simons, L., Elman, I., & Eccleston, C. (2018). When pain gets stuck: The evolution of pain chronification and treatment resistance. *Pain, 159*(12), 2421–2436.

Bowen, S., Witkiewitz, K., Dillworth, T. M., Chawla, N., Simpson, T. L., Ostafin, B. D., Larimer, M. E., Blume, A. W., Parks, G. A., & Marlatt, G. A. (2006). Mindfulness meditation and substance use in an incarcerated population. *Psychology of Addictive Behaviors, 20*(3), 343–347.

Brickman, P., & Campbell, D. T. (1971). Hedonic relativism and planning the good science. In M. H. Appley (Ed.), *Adaptation level theory: A symposium* (pp. 287–302). Academic Press.

Brodal, P. (2004). *The central nervous system: Structure and function.* Oxford University Press.

Brown, K. W., Creswell, J. D., & Ryan, R. M. (2015). *Handbook of mindfulness: Theory, research, and practice.* Guilford Press.

Bryant, F. B., & Veroff, J. (2017). *Savoring: A new model of positive experience.* Psychology Press.

Buer, N., & Linton, S. J. (2002). Fear-avoidance beliefs and catastrophizing: Occurrence and risk factor in back pain and ADL in the general population. *Pain, 99*(3), 485–491.

Bushnell, M. C., Čeko, M., & Low, L. A. (2013). Cognitive and emotional control of pain and its disruption in chronic pain. *Nature Reviews Neuroscience, 14*(7), 502–511.

Butler, A. C., Chapman, J. E., Forman, E. M., & Beck, A. T. (2006). The empirical status of cognitive-behavioral therapy: A review of meta-analyses. *Clinical Psychology Review, 26,* 17–31.

Butler, S. F., Budman, S. H., Fernandez, K. C., Houle, B., Benoit, C., Katz, N., & Jamison, R. N. (2007). Development and validation of the current opioid misuse measure. *Pain, 130,* 144–156.

Campbell, C. M., Carroll, C. P., Kiley, K., Han, D., Haywood, C., Jr., Lanzkron, S., Swedberg, L., Edwards, R. R., Page, G. G., & Haythornthwaite, J. A. (2016). Quantitative sensory testing and pain-evoked cytokine reactivity: Comparison of patients with sickle cell disease to healthy matched controls. *Pain, 157*(4), 949–956.

Cannon, W. B. (1929). Organization of physiological homeostasis. *Physiology Review, 9*(3), 399–431.

Carpenter, J. K., Conroy, K., Gomez, A. F., Curren, L. C., & Hofmann, S. G. (2019). The relationship between trait mindfulness and affective symptoms: A meta-analysis of the Five Facet Mindfulness Questionnaire (FFMQ). *Clinical Psychology Review, 74,* 101785.

Carpenter, R. W., Lane, S. P., Bruehl, S., & Trull, T. J. (2019). Concurrent and lagged associations of prescription opioid use with pain and negative affect in the daily lives of chronic pain patients. *Journal of Consulting and Clinical Psychology, 87*(10), 872–886.

Carvalho, C., Caetano, J. M., Cunha, L., Rebouta, P., Kaptchuk, T. J., & Kirsch, I. (2016). Open-label placebo treatment in chronic low back pain: A randomized controlled trial. *Pain, 157*(12), 2766–2772.

Case, A., & Deaton, A. (2015). Rising morbidity and mortality in midlife among White non-Hispanic Americans in the 21st century. *Proceedings of the National Academy of Sciences, 112*(49), 15078–15083.

Centers for Disease Control and Prevention. (2020, December 17). *Increase in fatal drug overdoses across the United States driven by synthetic opioids before and during the COVID-19 pandemic.* HAN Archive–00438 | Health Alert Network (HAN). *https://emergency.cdc.gov/han/2020/han00438.asp*

Chapman, C. R., Tuckett, R. P., & Song, C. W. (2008). Pain and stress in a systems perspective: Reciprocal neural, endocrine, and immune interactions. *Journal of Pain, 9*(2), 122–145.

Chartrand, T. L., & Bargh, J. A. (1999). The chameleon effect: The perception–behavior link and social interaction. *Journal of Personality and Social Psychology, 76*(6), 893–910.

Chiara, G. D., & North, R. A. (1992). Neurobiology

of opiate abuse. *Trends in Pharmacological Sciences, 13,* 185–193.

Chou, R., Fanciullo, G. J., Fine, P. G., Adler, J. A., Ballantyne, J. C., Davies, P., Donovan, M. I., Fishbain, D. A., Foley, K. M., Fudin, J., Gilson, A. M., Kelter, A., Mauskop, A., O'Connor, P. G., Passik, S. D., Pasternak, G. W., Portenoy, R. K., Rich, B. A., Roberts, R. G., . . . American Pain Society–American Academy of Pain Medicine Opiods Guidelines Panel. (2009). Clinical guidelines for the use of chronic opioid therapy in chronic noncancer pain. *Journal of Pain, 10*(2), 113–130.

Chou, R., Turner, J. A., Devine, E. B., Hansen, R. N., Sullivan, S. D., Blazina, I., Dana, T., Bougatsos, C., & Deyo, R. A. (2015). The effectiveness and risks of long-term opioid therapy for chronic pain: A systematic review for a National Institutes of Health Pathways to Prevention Workshop. *Annals of Internal Medicine, 162*(4), 276–286.

Christie, M. J. (2008). Cellular neuroadaptations to chronic opioids: Tolerance, withdrawal and addiction. *British Journal of Pharmacology, 154*(2), 384–396.

Chu, L. F., Angst, M. S., & Clark, D. (2008). Opioid-induced hyperalgesia in humans: Molecular mechanisms and clinical considerations. *Clinical Journal of Pain, 24,* 479–496.

Colloca, L., & Barsky, A. J. (2020). Placebo and nocebo effects. *New England Journal of Medicine, 382*(6), 554–561.

Cooperman, N. A., Hanley, A. W., Kline, A., & Garland, E. L. (2021). A pilot randomized clinical trial of mindfulness-oriented recovery enhancement as an adjunct to methadone treatment for people with opioid use disorder and chronic pain: Impact on illicit drug use, health, and well-being. *Journal of Substance Abuse Treatment,* 108468.

Cooperman, N. A., Lu, S. E., Hanley, A. W., Puvananayagam, T., Dooley-Budsock, P., Kline, A., & Garland, E. L. (2023). Telehealth Mindfulness-Oriented Recovery Enhancement vs usual care in individuals with opioid use disorder and pain: A randomized clinical trial. *JAMA Psychiatry.*

Covey, S. R. (2010). Foreword. In A. Pattakos (Ed.), *Prisoners of our thoughts: Viktor Frankl's principles for discovering meaning in life and work* (2nd ed., pp. v–xi). Berrett-Koehler.

Craig, A. D. (2003). Interoception: The sense of the physiological condition of the body. *Current Opinion in Neurobiology, 13,* 500–505.

Crombez, G., Van Damme, S., & Eccleston, C.

(2005). Hypervigilance to pain: An experimental and clinical analysis. *Pain, 116*(1), 4–7.

Dahlhamer, J., Lucas, J., Zelaya, C., Nahin, R., Mackey, S., DeBar, L., Kerns, R., Von Korff, M., Porter, L., & Helmick, C. (2018). Prevalence of chronic pain and high-impact chronic pain among adults—United States, 2016. *Morbidity and Mortality Weekly Report, 67*(36), 1001–1006.

Dakwar, E., Nunes, E. V., Hart, C. L., Hu, M. C., Foltin, R. W., & Levin, F. R. (2018). A sub-set of psychoactive effects may be critical to the behavioral impact of ketamine on cocaine use disorder: Results from a randomized, controlled laboratory study. *Neuropharmacology, 142*, 270–276.

Darnall, B. D., & Fields, H. L. (2022). Clinical and neuroscience evidence supports the critical importance of patient expectations and agency in opioid tapering. *Pain, 163*(5), 824–826.

Davidson, R. J., Kabat-Zinn, J., Schumacher, J., Rosenkranz, M., Muller, D., Santorelli, S. F., Urbanowski, F., Harrington, A., Bonus, K., & Sheridan, J. F. (2003). Alterations in brain and immune function produced by mindfulness meditation. *Psychosomatic Medicine, 65*(4), 564–570.

de Shazer, S. (1988). *Clues: Investigating solutions in brief therapy.* Norton.

de Wied, M., & Verbaten, M. N. (2001). Affective pictures processing, attention, and pain tolerance. *Pain, 90*(1–2), 163–172.

Deegan, P. E. (1997). Recovery and empowerment for people with psychiatric disabilities. *Social Work in Health Care, 25*(3), 11–24.

Deikman, A. J. (1966). Deautomatization and the mystic experience. *Psychiatry, 29*, 324–388.

Delorme, J., Kerckhove, N., Authier, N., Pereira, B., Bertin, C., & Chenaf, C. (2023). Systematic review and meta-analysis of the prevalence of chronic pain among patients with opioid use disorder and receiving opioid substitution therapy. *Journal of Pain, 24*(2), 192–203.

Depraz, N., Varela, F., & Vermersch, P. (2003). *On becoming aware: A pragmatics of experiencing.* John Benjamins.

Desimone, R., & Duncan, J. (1995). Neural mechanisms of selective visual attention. *Annual Review of Neuroscience, 18*, 193–222.

Deutsch, E., & Dalvi, R. (2004). *The essential Vedānta: A new source book of Advaita Vedānta.* World Wisdom.

Dimsdale, J. E., & Dantzer, R. (2007). A biological substrate for somatoform disorders: Importance of pathophysiology. *Psychosomatic Medicine, 69*(9), 850–854.

Dismore, L., van Wersch, A., Critchley, R., Aradhyula, A. M., & Swainston, K. (2020). The associations of pain catastrophizing and postoperative outcomes in domains of pain, quality of life, and function in joint replacement surgery: A systematic review. *Journal of Pain Management, 13*(2), 105–113.

Dogen, E. (2010). *Dogen's extensive record: A translation of the Eihei Koroku.* Simon & Schuster.

Doré, B. P., Boccagno, C., Burr, D., Hubbard, A., Long, K., Weber, J., Stern, Y., & Ochsner, K. N. (2017). Finding positive meaning in negative experiences engages ventral striatal and ventromedial prefrontal regions associated with reward valuation. *Journal of Cognitive Neuroscience, 29*(2), 235–244.

Dormandy, T. (2012). *Opium: Reality's dark dream.* Yale University Press.

Dowell, D., Haegerich, T. M., & Chou, R. (2016). CDC guideline for prescribing opioids for chronic pain—United States, 2016. *JAMA, 315*(15), 1624–1645.

Dubin, A. E., & Patapoutian, A. (2010). Nociceptors: The sensors of the pain pathway. *Journal of Clinical Investigation, 120*(11), 3760–3772.

Dunne, J. (2011). Toward an understanding of nondual mindfulness. *Contemporary Buddhism, 12*(1), 71–88.

Dunne, J. D., Thompson, E., & Schooler, J. (2019). Mindful meta-awareness: Sustained and nonpropositional. *Current Opinion in Psychology, 28*, 307–311.

Dyczkowski, M. S. (1987). *The doctrine of vibration: An analysis of the doctrines and practices associated with Kashmir Shaivism.* SUNY Press.

Dyczkowski, M. S. (1992). *The aphorisms of Siva: The Siva Sutra with Bhaskara's commentary, the Varttika.* SUNY Press.

Eccleston, C., & Crombez, G. (1999). Pain demands attention: A cognitive–affective model of the interruptive function of pain. *Psychological Bulletin, 125*(3), 356–366.

Edwards, R. R., Dworkin, R. H., Sullivan, M. D., Turk, D. C., & Wasan, A. D. (2016). The role of psychosocial processes in the development and maintenance of chronic pain. *Journal of Pain, 17*(9), T70–T92.

Edwards, R. R., Kronfli, T., Haythornthwaite, J. A., Smith, M. T., McGuire, L., & Page, G. G. (2008). Association of catastrophizing with interleukin-6 responses to acute pain. *Pain, 140*(1), 135–144.

Egan, R. P., Hill, K. E., & Foti, D. (2017). Differential

effects of state and trait mindfulness on the late positive potential. *Emotion, 18*(8), 1128–1141.

Engel, G. L. (1977). The need for a new medical model: A challenge for biomedicine. *Science, 196,* 129–136.

Erickson, M. H., Rossi, E. L., & Rossi, S. (1976). *Hypnotic realities: The induction of clinical hypnosis and forms of indirect suggestion.* Irvington.

Everitt, B. J., & Robbins, T. W. (2016). Drug addiction: Updating actions to habits to compulsions ten years on. *Annual Review of Psychology, 67,* 23–50.

Fabbro, A., Crescentini, C., Matiz, A., Clarici, A., & Fabbro, F. (2017). Effects of mindfulness meditation on conscious and non-conscious components of the mind. *Applied Sciences, 7*(4), 349.

Feldman, C., & Kuyken, W. (2011). Compassion in the landscape of suffering. *Contemporary Buddhism, 12*(1), 143–155.

Feldman, G. C., Joormann, J., & Johnson, S. L. (2008). Responses to positive affect: A self-report measure of rumination and dampening. *Cognitive Therapy and Research, 32*(4), 507.

Field, M., & Cox, W. (2008). Attentional bias in addictive behaviors: A review of its development, causes, and consequences. *Drug and Alcohol Dependence, 97*(1–2), 1–20.

Field, M., Munafò, M. R., & Franken, I. H. (2009). A meta-analytic investigation of the relationship between attentional bias and subjective craving in substance abuse. *Psychological Bulletin, 135*(4), 589–607.

Fields, H. (2004). State-dependent opioid control of pain. *Nature Reviews Neuroscience, 5*(7), 565–575.

Fields, H. L. (2011). Mu opioid receptor mediated analgesia and reward. In G. Pasternak (Ed.), *The opiate receptors: The receptors* (pp. 239–264). Humana Press.

Finan, P., Hunt, C., Keaser, M., Lerman, S., Smith, K., Bingham, C., Barrett, F., Zeidan, F., Garland, E. L. & Seminowicz, D. (2022). Effects of savoring meditation on pain-related corticostriatal and positive emotional function. *Journal of Pain, 23*(5), 32–33.

Flor, H., Turk, D. C., & Birbaumer, N. (1985). Assessment of stress-related psychophysiological reactions in chronic back pain patients. *Journal of Consulting and Clinical Psychology, 53*(3), 354–364.

Fox, K. C., Nijeboer, S., Dixon, M. L., Floman, J. L., Ellamil, M., Rumak, S. P., Sedlmeier, P., & Christoff, K. (2014). Is meditation associated with altered brain structure? A systematic review and meta-analysis of morphometric neuroimaging in meditation practitioners. *Neuroscience and Biobehavioral Reviews, 43,* 48–73.

Frankl, V. E. (1959). *Man's search for meaning.* Simon & Schuster. (Original work published 1946)

Froeliger, B., Garland, E. L., Kozink, R. V., Modlin, L. A., Chen, N.-K., McClernon, F. J., Greeson, J. M., & Sobin, P. (2012). Meditation-state functional connectivity (MSFC): Strengthening of the dorsal attention network and beyond. *Evidence-Based Complementary and Alternative Medicine, 2012,* 680407.

Froeliger, B., Mathew, A. R., McConnell, P. A., Eichberg, C., Saladin, M. E., Carpenter, M. J., & Garland, E. L. (2017). Restructuring reward mechanisms in nicotine addiction: A pilot fMRI study of mindfulness-oriented recovery enhancement for cigarette smokers. *Evidence-Based Complementary and Alternative Medicine, 2017,* e7018014.

Froese, T., Gould, C., & Barrett, A. (2011). Reviewing from within a commentary on first- and second-person methods in the science of consciousness. *Constructivist Foundations, 6*(2), 254–269.

Garfield, J. B., Lubman, D. I., & Yücel, M. (2014). Anhedonia in substance use disorders: A systematic review of its nature, course and clinical correlates. *Australian and New Zealand Journal of Psychiatry, 48*(1), 36–51.

Garland, E. L. (2011). Trait mindfulness predicts attentional and autonomic regulation of alcohol cue-reactivity. *Journal of Psychophysiology, 25*(4), 180–189.

Garland, E. L. (2013). *Mindfulness-oriented recovery enhancement for addiction, stress, and pain.* NASW Press.

Garland, E. L. (2016). Restructuring reward processing with mindfulness-oriented recovery enhancement: Novel therapeutic mechanisms to remediate hedonic dysregulation in addiction, stress, and pain. *Annals of the New York Academy of Sciences, 1373*(1), 25–37.

Garland, E. L. (2020). Psychosocial intervention and the reward system in pain and opioid misuse: New opportunities and directions. *Pain, 161*(12), 2659–2666.

Garland, E. L. (2021). Mindful positive emotion regulation as a treatment for addiction: From hedonic pleasure to self-transcendent meaning. *Current Opinion in Behavioral Sciences, 39,* 168–177.

Garland, E. L., Atchley, R. M., Hanley, A. W.,

Zubieta, J.-K., & Froeliger, B. (2019). Mindfulness-oriented recovery enhancement remediates hedonic dysregulation in opioid users: Neural and affective evidence of target engagement. *Science Advances, 5*(10), eaax1569.

Garland, E. L., Baker, A. K., & Howard, M. O. (2017). Mindfulness-oriented recovery enhancement reduces opioid attentional bias among prescription opioid-treated chronic pain patients. *Journal of the Society for Social Work and Research, 8*(4), 493–509.

Garland, E. L., Boettiger, C. A., Gaylord, S., Chanon, V. W., & Howard, M. O. (2012). Mindfulness is inversely associated with alcohol attentional bias among recovering alcohol-dependent adults. *Cognitive Therapy and Research, 36*(5), 441–450.

Garland, E. L., Brown, S. M., & Howard, M. O. (2016). Thought suppression as a mediator of the association between depressed mood and prescription opioid craving among chronic pain patients. *Journal of Behavioral Medicine, 39*(1), 128–138.

Garland, E. L., Bryan, C. J., Finan, P. H., Thomas, E. A., Priddy, S. E., Riquino, M. R., & Howard, M. O. (2017). Pain, hedonic regulation, and opioid misuse: Modulation of momentary experience by mindfulness-oriented recovery enhancement in opioid-treated chronic pain patients. *Drug and Alcohol Dependence, 173*, S65–S72.

Garland, E. L., Bryan, C. J., Kreighbaum, L., Nakamura, Y., Howard, M. O., & Froeliger, B. (2018). Prescription opioid misusing chronic pain patients exhibit dysregulated context-dependent associations: Investigating associative learning in addiction with the cue-primed reactivity task. *Drug and Alcohol Dependence, 187*, 13–21.

Garland, E. L., Bryan, C. J., Nakamura, Y., Froeliger, B., & Howard, M. O. (2017). Deficits in autonomic indices of emotion regulation and reward processing associated with prescription opioid use and misuse. *Psychopharmacology, 234*(4), 621–629.

Garland, E. L., Bryan, M. A., Priddy, S. E., Riquino, M. R., Froeliger, B., & Howard, M. O. (2019). Effects of mindfulness-oriented recovery enhancement versus social support on negative affective interference during inhibitory control among opioid-treated chronic pain patients: A pilot mechanistic study. *Annals of Behavioral Medicine, 53*(10), 865–876.

Garland, E. L., Farb, N. A., Goldin, P. R., & Fredrickson, B. L. (2015a). Mindfulness broadens awareness and builds eudaimonic meaning: A process model of mindful positive emotion regulation. *Psychological Inquiry, 26*(4), 293–314.

Garland, E. L., Farb, N. A., Goldin, P. R., & Fredrickson, B. L. (2015b). The mindfulness-to-meaning theory: Extensions, applications, and challenges at the attention–appraisal–emotion interface. *Psychological Inquiry, 26*(4), 377–387.

Garland, E. L., Fix, S. T., Hudak, J. P., Bernat, E. M., Nakamura, Y., Hanley, A. W., Donaldson, G. W., Marchand, W. R., & Froeliger, B. (2023). Mindfulness-oriented recovery enhancement remediates anhedonia in chronic opioid use by enhancing neurophysiological responses during savoring of natural rewards. *Psychological Medicine, 53*(5), 2085–2094.

Garland, E. L., & Fredrickson, B. L. (2019). Positive psychological states in the arc from mindfulness to self-transcendence: Extensions of the mindfulness-to-meaning theory and applications to addiction and chronic pain treatment. *Current Opinion in Psychology, 28*, 184–191.

Garland, E. L., Fredrickson, B. L., Kring, A. M., Johnson, D. P., Meyer, P. S., & Penn, D. L. (2010). Upward spirals of positive emotions counter downward spirals of negativity: Insights from the broaden-and-build theory and affective neuroscience on the treatment of emotion dysfunctions and deficits in psychopathology. *Clinical Psychology Review, 30*, 849–864.

Garland, E. L., Froeliger, B., & Howard, M. O. (2013). Mindfulness training targets neurocognitive mechanisms of addiction at the attention–appraisal–emotion interface. *Frontiers in Psychiatry, 4*, 173.

Garland, E. L., Froeliger, B., & Howard, M. O. (2014). Effects of mindfulness-oriented recovery enhancement on reward responsiveness and opioid cue-reactivity. *Psychopharmacology, 231*(16), 3229–3238.

Garland, E. L., Froeliger, B., & Howard, M. O. (2015a). Allostatic dysregulation of natural reward processing in prescription opioid misuse: Autonomic and attentional evidence. *Biological Psychology, 105*, 124–129.

Garland, E. L., Froeliger, B., & Howard, M. O. (2015b). Neurophysiological evidence for remediation of reward processing deficits in chronic pain and opioid misuse following treatment with mindfulness-oriented recovery enhancement: Exploratory ERP findings from a pilot RCT. *Journal of Behavioral Medicine, 38*(2), 327–336.

Garland, E. L., Froeliger, B. E., Passik, S. D., &

Howard, M. O. (2013). Attentional bias for prescription opioid cues among opioid dependent chronic pain patients. *Journal of Behavioral Medicine, 36*(6), 611–620.

Garland, E. L., Froeliger, B., Zeidan, F., Partin, K., & Howard, M. O. (2013). The downward spiral of chronic pain, prescription opioid misuse, and addiction: Cognitive, affective, and neuropsychopharmacologic pathways. *Neuroscience and Biobehavioral Reviews, 37*(10), 2597–2607.

Garland, E. L., Gaylord, S. A., & Fredrickson, B. L. (2011). Positive reappraisal mediates the stress-reductive effects of mindfulness: An upward spiral process. *Mindfulness, 2*, 59–67.

Garland, E. L., Gaylord, S. A., Palsson, O., Faurot, K., Mann, J. D., & Whitehead, W. E. (2012). Therapeutic mechanisms of a mindfulness-based treatment for IBS: Effects on visceral sensitivity, catastrophizing, and affective processing of pain sensations. *Journal of Behavioral Medicine, 35*(6), 591–602.

Garland, E. L., Gaylord, S. A., & Park, J. (2009). The role of mindfulness in positive reappraisal. *Explore (NY), 5*, 37–44.

Garland, E. L., Hanley, A. W., Bedford, C. E., Zubieta, J.-K., Howard, M. O., Nakamura, Y., Donaldson, G. W., & Froeliger, B. (2018). Reappraisal deficits promote craving and emotional distress among chronic pain patients at risk for prescription opioid misuse. *Journal of Addictive Diseases*, 1–9.

Garland, E. L., Hanley, A. W., Hudak, J., Nakamura, Y., & Froeliger, B. (2022). Mindfulness-induced endogenous theta stimulation occasions self-transcendence and inhibits addictive behavior. *Science Advances, 8*(41), eabo4455.

Garland, E. L., Hanley, A. W., Kline, A., & Cooperman, N. A. (2019). Mindfulness-oriented recovery enhancement reduces opioid craving among individuals with opioid use disorder and chronic pain in medication assisted treatment: Ecological momentary assessments from a stage 1 randomized controlled trial. *Drug and Alcohol Dependence, 203*(1), 61–65.

Garland, E. L., Hanley, A. W., Nakamura, Y., Barrett, J. W., Baker, A. K., Reese, S. E., Riquino, M. R., Froeliger, B., & Donaldson, G. W. (2022). Mindfulness-oriented recovery enhancement vs supportive group therapy for co-occurring opioid misuse and chronic pain in primary care: A randomized clinical trial. *JAMA Internal Medicine, 182*(4), 407–417.

Garland, E. L., Hanley, A. W., Riquino, M. R.,

Reese, S. E., Baker, A. K., Salas, K., Yack, B. P., Bedford, C. E., Bryan, M. A., Atchley, R., Nakamura, Y., Froeliger, B., & Howard, M. O. (2019). Mindfulness-oriented recovery enhancement reduces opioid misuse risk via analgesic and positive psychological mechanisms: A randomized controlled trial. *Journal of Consulting and Clinical Psychology, 87*(10), 927–940.

Garland, E. L., & Howard, M. O. (2009). Neuroplasticity, psychosocial genomics, and the biopsychosocial paradigm in the 21st century. *Health and Social Work, 34*, 191–200.

Garland, E. L., & Howard, M. O. (2013). Mindfulness-oriented recovery enhancement reduces pain attentional bias in chronic pain patients. *Psychotherapy and Psychosomatics, 82*(5), 311–318.

Garland, E. L., & Howard, M. O. (2014). Opioid attentional bias and cue-elicited craving predict future risk of prescription opioid misuse among chronic pain patients. *Drug and Alcohol Dependence, 144*, 283–287.

Garland, E. L., Howard, M. O., Zubieta, J. K., & Froeliger, B. (2017). Restructuring hedonic dysregulation in chronic pain and prescription opioid misuse: Effects of mindfulness-oriented recovery enhancement on responsiveness to drug cues and natural rewards. *Psychotherapy and Psychosomatics, 86*(2), 111–112.

Garland, E. L., Hudak, J., Hanley, A. W., & Nakamura, Y. (2020). Mindfulness-oriented recovery enhancement reduces opioid dose in primary care by strengthening autonomic regulation during meditation. *American Psychologist, 75*(6), 840–852.

Garland, E. L., Kiken, L. G., Faurot, K., Palsson, O., & Gaylord, S. A. (2017). Upward spirals of mindfulness and reappraisal: Testing the mindfulness-to-meaning theory with autoregressive latent trajectory modeling. *Cognitive Therapy and Research, 41*(3), 381–392.

Garland, E. L., Nakamura, Y., Bryan, C. J., Hanley, A. W., Parisi, A., Froeliger, B., Marchand, W. R., & Donaldson, G. W. (2024). Mindfulness-oriented recovery enhancement for veterans and military personnel on long-term opioid therapy for chronic pain: A randomized clinical trial. *American Journal of Psychiatry, 181*(2), 125–134.

Garland, E. L., Reese, S. E., Bedford, C. E., & Baker, A. K. (2019). Adverse childhood experiences predict autonomic indices of emotion dysregulation and negative emotional cue-elicited craving among female opioid-treated chronic pain patients. *Development and Psychopathology, 31*(3), 1101–1110.

Garland, E. L., Roberts-Lewis, A., Tronnier, C. D., Graves, R., & Kelley, K. (2016). Mindfulness-Oriented Recovery Enhancement versus CBT for co-occurring substance dependence, traumatic stress, and psychiatric disorders: Proximal outcomes from a pragmatic randomized trial. *Behaviour Research and Therapy, 77*, 7–16.

Garland, E. L., Trøstheim, M., Eikemo, M., Ernst, G., & Leknes, S. (2020). Anhedonia in chronic pain and prescription opioid misuse. *Psychological Medicine, 50*(12), 1977–1988.

Geneen, L. J., Moore, R. A., Clarke, C., Martin, D., Colvin, L. A., & Smith, B. H. (2017). Physical activity and exercise for chronic pain in adults: An overview of Cochrane Reviews. *Cochrane Database of Systematic Reviews, 4*, CD011279.

Geschwind, N., Peeters, F., Drukker, M., van Os, J., & Wichers, M. (2011). Mindfulness training increases momentary positive emotions and reward experience in adults vulnerable to depression: A randomized controlled trial. *Journal of Consulting and Clinical Psychology, 79*(5), 618–628.

Goldin, P. R., Thurston, M., Allende, S., Moodie, C., Dixon, M. L., Heimberg, R. G., & Gross, J. J. (2021). Evaluation of cognitive behavioral therapy vs mindfulness meditation in brain changes during reappraisal and acceptance among patients with social anxiety disorder: A randomized clinical trial. *JAMA Psychiatry, 78*(10), 1134–1142.

Goleman, D., & Davidson, R. J. (2018). *Altered traits: Science reveals how meditation changes your mind, brain, and body.* Penguin.

Goyal, M., Singh, S., Sibinga, E. M. S., Gould, N. F., Rowland-Seymour, A., Sharma, R., Berger, Z., Sleicher, D., Maron, D. D., Shihab, H. M., Ranasinghe, P. D., Linn, S., Saha, S., Bass, E. B., & Haythornthwaite, J. A. (2014). Meditation programs for psychological stress and well-being: A systematic review and meta-analysis. *JAMA Internal Medicine, 174*(3), 357–368.

Greenberg, J., Reiner, K., & Meiran, N. (2012). "Mind the trap": Mindfulness practice reduces cognitive rigidity. *PLOS ONE, 7*(5), e36206.

Griffiths, R. R., Johnson, M. W., Carducci, M. A., Umbricht, A., Richards, W. A., Richards, B. D., Cosimano, M. P., & Klinedinst, M. A. (2016). Psilocybin produces substantial and sustained decreases in depression and anxiety in patients with life-threatening cancer: A randomized

double-blind trial. *Journal of Psychopharmacology, 30*(12), 1181–1197.

Grinder, J., DeLozier, J., & Bandler, R. (1977). *Patterns of the hypnotic techniques of Milton H. Erickson, M.D.* (Vol. II). Metamorphous Press.

Gu, J., Strauss, C., Bond, R., & Cavanagh, K. (2015). How do mindfulness-based cognitive therapy and mindfulness-based stress reduction improve mental health and wellbeing? A systematic review and meta-analysis of mediation studies. *Clinical Psychology Review, 37*, 1–12.

Hadjistavropoulos, T., Craig, K. D., & Fuchs-Lacelle, S. (2004). Social influences and the communication of pain. In T. Hadjistavropoulos & K. D. Craig (Eds.), *Pain: Psychological perspectives* (pp. 87–112). Erlbaum.

Hagerty, M. R., Isaacs, J., Brasington, L., Shupe, L., Fetz, E. E., & Cramer, S. C. (2013). Case study of ecstatic meditation: FMRI and EEG evidence of self-stimulating a reward system. *Neural Plasticity, 2013*, 653572.

Han, B., Compton, W. M., Blanco, C., Crane, E., Lee, J., & Jones, C. M. (2017). Prescription opioid use, misuse, and use disorders in U.S. adults: 2015 National Survey on Drug Use and Health. *Annals of Internal Medicine, 167*(5), 293–301.

Hanh, T. N. (1988). *The sun my heart.* Parallax Press.

Hanley, A. W., & Garland, E. L. (2019a). Mapping the affective dimension of embodiment with the sensation manikin: Validation among chronic pain patients and modification by mindfulness-oriented recovery enhancement. *Psychosomatic Medicine, 81*(7), 612–621.

Hanley, A. W., & Garland, E. L. (2019b). Mindfulness training disrupts Pavlovian conditioning. *Physiology and Behavior, 204*, 151–154.

Hanley, A. W., & Garland, E. L. (2021). The Mindfulness-Oriented Recovery Enhancement Fidelity Measure (MORE-FM): Development and validation of a new tool to assess therapist adherence and competence. *Journal of Evidence-Based Social Work, 18*(3), 308–322.

Hanley, A. W., & Garland, E. L. (2022). Self-transcendence predicts better pre- and postoperative outcomes in two randomized clinical trials of brief mindfulness-based interventions. *Mindfulness, 13*(6), 1532–1543.

Hanley, A. W., Gililland, J., & Garland, E. L. (2021). To be mindful of the breath or pain: Comparing two brief preoperative mindfulness techniques for total joint arthroplasty patients. *Journal of Consulting and Clinical Psychology, 89*(7), 590–600.

Hanley, A. W., Nakamura, Y., & Garland, E. L. (2018). The Nondual Awareness Dimensional Assessment (NADA): New tools to assess nondual traits and states of consciousness occurring within and beyond the context of meditation. *Psychological Assessment*, 30(12), 1625–1639.

Hashmi, J. A., Baliki, M. N., Huang, L., Baria, A. T., Torbey, S., Hermann, K. M., Schnitzer, T. J., & Apkarian, A. V. (2013). Shape shifting pain: Chronification of back pain shifts brain representation from nociceptive to emotional circuits. *Brain*, 136(9), 2751–2768.

Haythornthwaite, J. A., Menefee, L. A., Heinberg, L. J., & Clark, M. R. (1998). Pain coping strategies predict perceived control over pain. *Pain*, 77(1), 33–39.

Hoehl, S., Fairhurst, M., & Schirmer, A. (2021). Interactional synchrony: Signals, mechanisms and benefits. *Social Cognitive and Affective Neuroscience*, 16(1–2), 5–18.

Hollins, M., Harper, D., Gallagher, S., Owings, E. W., Lim, P. F., Miller, V., Siddiqi, M. Q., & Maixner, W. (2009). Perceived intensity and unpleasantness of cutaneous and auditory stimuli: An evaluation of the generalized hypervigilance hypothesis. *Pain*, 141(3), 215–221.

Holzel, B. K., Carmody, J., Vangel, M., Congleton, C., Yerramsetti, S. M., Gard, T., & Lazar, S. W. (2011). Mindfulness practice leads to increases in regional brain gray matter density. *Psychiatry Research*, 191, 36–43.

Homer. (1946). *The Odyssey* (E. V. Rieu, Trans.). Penguin Books. (Original work published ca. 700 B.C.E.)

Huang, Y., Ceceli, A.O., Kronberg, G., King, S., Malaker, P., Alia-Klein, N., Garland, E.L., & Goldstein, R.Z. (2024). Association of corticostriatal engagement during cue-reactivity, reappraisal, and savoring of drug and non-drug stimuli with craving in heroin addiction. *American Journal of Psychiatry*, 181(2), 153–165.

Hudak, J., Bernat, E. M., Fix, S. T., Prince, K. C., Froeliger, B., & Garland, E. L. (2022). Neurophysiological deficits during reappraisal of negative emotional stimuli in opioid misuse. *Biological Psychiatry*, 91(12), 1070–1078.

Hudak, J., Hanley, A. W., Marchand, W. R., Nakamura, Y., Yabko, B., & Garland, E. L. (2021). Endogenous theta stimulation during meditation predicts reduced opioid dosing following treatment with mindfulness-oriented recovery enhancement. *Neuropsychopharmacology*, 46(4), 836–843.

Huhn, A. S., Brooner, R. K., Sweeney, M. M., Antoine, D., Hammond, A. S., Ayaz, H., & Dunn, K. E. (2021). The association of prefrontal cortex response during a natural reward cue-reactivity paradigm, anhedonia, and demoralization in persons maintained on methadone. *Addictive Behaviors*, 113, 106673.

Ives, T. J., Chelminski, P. R., Hammett-Stabler, C. A., Malone, R. M., Perhac, J. S., Potisek, N. M., Shilliday, B. B., DeWalt, D. A., & Pignone, M. P. (2006). Predictors of opioid misuse in patients with chronic pain: A prospective cohort study. *BMC Health Services Research*, 6(1), 46.

Jamison, R. N., Martel, M. O., Huang, C.-C., Jurcik, D., & Edwards, R. R. (2016). Efficacy of the Opioid Compliance Checklist to monitor chronic pain patients receiving opioid therapy in primary care. *Journal of Pain*, 17(4), 414–423.

Jansen, J. E., Gleeson, J., Bendall, S., Rice, S., & Alvarez-Jimenez, M. (2020). Acceptance- and mindfulness-based interventions for persons with psychosis: A systematic review and meta-analysis. *Schizophrenia Research*, 215, 25–37.

Jastrzab, L., Mackey, S., Chu, L., Stringer, E., & Younger, J. (2012). Neural correlates of opioid induced hyperalgesia. *Journal of Pain*, 13(4), S51.

John, W. S., & Wu, L.-T. (2020). Chronic noncancer pain among adults with substance use disorders: Prevalence, characteristics, and association with opioid overdose and healthcare utilization. *Drug and Alcohol Dependence*, 209, 107902.

Johnson, S. W., & North, R. A. (1992). Opioids excite dopamine neurons by hyperpolarization of local interneurons. *Journal of Neuroscience*, 12(2), 483–488.

Josipovic, Z. (2014). Neural correlates of nondual awareness in meditation. *Annals of the New York Academy of Sciences*, 1307(1), 9–18.

Julien, R. M. (2007). *A primer of drug action: A comprehensive guide to the actions, uses, and side effects of psychoactive drugs* (11th ed.). Worth.

Julius, D., & Basbaum, A. I. (2001). Molecular mechanisms of nociception. *Nature*, 413(685), 203–210.

Kabat-Zinn, J. (1982). An outpatient program in behavioral medicine for chronic pain patients based on the practice of mindfulness meditation: Theoretical considerations and preliminary results. *General Hospital Psychiatry*, 4(1), 33–47.

Kabat-Zinn, J. (1990). *Full catastrophe living: Using the wisdom of your body and mind to face stress, pain, and illness*. Delacorte Press.

Kabat-Zinn, J. (2003). Mindfulness-based interventions in context: Past, present, and future. *Clinical Psychology: Science and Practice, 10,* 144–156.

Kabat-Zinn, J. (2005). *Coming to our senses: Healing ourselves and the world through mindfulness.* Hachette Books.

Kabat-Zinn, J. (2011). Some reflections on the origins of MBSR, skillful means, and the trouble with maps. *Contemporary Buddhism, 12,* 281–306.

Kabat-Zinn, J. (2019). Foreword: Seeds of a necessary global renaissance in the making—The refining of psychology's understanding of the nature of mind, self, and embodiment through the lens of mindfulness and its origins at a key inflection point for the species. *Current Opinion in Psychology, 28,* xi–xvii.

Kalivas, P. W., & O'Brien, C. (2008). Drug addiction as a pathology of staged neuroplasticity. *Neuropsychopharmacology, 33*(1), 166–180.

Karyadi, K. A., VanderVeen, J. D., & Cyders, M. A. (2014). A meta-analysis of the relationship between trait mindfulness and substance use behaviors. *Drug and Alcohol Dependence, 143*(Suppl. C), 1–10.

Kaul, M. (2020). Abhinavagupta on reflection (Pratibimba) in the Tantrāloka. *Journal of Indian Philosophy, 48*(2), 161–189.

Keefe, F. J., Wilkins, R. H., & Cook, W. A. (1984). Direct observation of pain behavior in low back pain patients during physical examination. *Pain, 20*(1), 59–68.

Keefe, P. R. (2021). *Empire of pain: The secret history of the Sackler dynasty.* Anchor.

Kelsen, B. A., Sumich, A., Kasabov, N., Liang, S. H. Y., & Wang, G. Y. (2020). What has social neuroscience learned from hyperscanning studies of spoken communication? A systematic review. *Neuroscience and Biobehavioral Reviews, 132,* 1249–1262.

Keogh, E., Ellery, D., Hunt, C., & Hannent, I. (2001). Selective attentional bias for pain-related stimuli amongst pain fearful individuals. *Pain, 91,* 91–100.

Kiken, L. G., Garland, E. L., Bluth, K., Palsson, O. S., & Gaylord, S. A. (2015). From a state to a trait: Trajectories of state mindfulness in meditation during intervention predict changes in trait mindfulness. *Personality and Individual Differences, 81,* 41–46.

Kirwilliam, S. S., & Derbyshire, S. W. G. (2008). Increased bias to report heat or pain following emotional priming of pain-related fear. *Pain, 137*(1), 60–65.

Klenerman, L., Slade, P. D., Stanley, I. M., Pennie, B., Reilly, J. P., Atchison, L. E., Troup, J. D., & Rose, M. J. (1995). The prediction of chronicity in patients with an acute attack of low back pain in a general practice setting. *Spine, 20*(4), 478–484.

Kober, H., Mende-Siedlecki, P., Kross, E. F., Weber, J., Mischel, W., Hart, C. L., & Ochsner, K. N. (2010). Prefrontal–striatal pathway underlies cognitive regulation of craving. *Proceedings of the National Academy of Sciences, 107*(33), 14811–14816.

Koob, G. F. (2020). Neurobiology of opioid addiction: Opponent process, hyperkatifeia, and negative reinforcement. *Biological Psychiatry, 87*(1), 44–53.

Koob, G. F., & Le Moal, M. (1997). Drug abuse: Hedonic homeostatic dysregulation. *Science, 278*(5335), 52–58.

Koob, G. F., & Le Moal, M. (2001). Drug addiction, dysregulation of reward, and allostasis. *Neuropsychopharmacology, 24*(2), 97–129.

Koob, G. F., & Volkow, N. D. (2016). Neurobiology of addiction: A neurocircuitry analysis. *Lancet Psychiatry, 3*(8), 760–773.

Kral, T. R. A., Davis, K., Korponay, C., Hirshberg, M. J., Hoel, R., Tello, L. Y., Goldman, R. I., Rosenkranz, M. A., Lutz, A., & Davidson, R. J. (2022). Absence of structural brain changes from mindfulness-based stress reduction: Two combined randomized controlled trials. *Science Advances, 8*(20), eabk3316.

Lama, D., & Vreeland, N. (Ed.). (2001). *An open heart: Practicing compassion in everyday life.* Little Brown.

Laozi, & English, J. (2011). *Tao te ching.* Vintage Books.

Lazarus, R. S., & Folkman, S. (1984). *Stress, appraisal, and coping.* Springer.

Le Merrer, J., Becker, J. A. J., Befort, K., & Kieffer, B. L. (2009). Reward processing by the opioid system in the brain. *Physiological Reviews, 89*(4), 1379–1412.

LeDoux, J. (2003). The emotional brain, fear, and the amygdala. *Cellular and Molecular Neurobiology, 23*(4), 727–738.

Lee, M. C., Wanigasekera, V., & Tracey, I. (2014). Imaging opioid analgesia in the human brain and its potential relevance for understanding opioid use in chronic pain. *Neuropharmacology, 84,* 123–130.

Legrain, V., Perchet, C., & García-Larrea, L. (2009). Involuntary orienting of attention to nociceptive events: Neural and behavioral signatures. *Journal of Neurophysiology*, *102*(4), 2423–2434.

Leighton, T. D. (2004). *The art of just sitting: Essential writings on the Zen practice of Shikantaza*. Simon & Schuster.

Leppä, M., Korvenoja, A., Carlson, S., Timonen, P., Martinkauppi, S., Ahonen, J., Rosenberg, P. H., Aronen, H. J., & Kalso, E. (2006). Acute opioid effects on human brain as revealed by functional magnetic resonance imaging. *NeuroImage*, *31*(2), 661–669.

Lewis, M. E., Pert, A., Pert, C. B., & Herkenham, M. (1983). Opiate receptor localization in rat cerebral cortex. *Journal of Comparative Neurology*, *216*(3), 339–358.

Leyland, A., Rowse, G., & Emerson, L.-M. (2019). Experimental effects of mindfulness inductions on self-regulation: Systematic review and meta-analysis. *Emotion*, *19*(1), 108–122.

Li, W., Howard, M. O., Garland, E. L., McGovern, P., & Lazar, M. (2017). Mindfulness treatment for substance misuse: A systematic review and meta-analysis. *Journal of Substance Abuse Treatment*, *75*, 62–96.

Linton, S. J., Buer, N., Vlaeyen, J., & Hellsing, A. L. (2000). Are fear-avoidance beliefs related to the inception of an episode of back pain? A prospective study. *Psychology and Health*, *14*(6), 1051–1059.

Loeser, J. D., & Melzack, R. (1999). Pain: An overview. *Lancet*, *353*(9164), 1607–1609.

Loggia, M. L., Kim, J., Gollub, R. L., Vangel, M. G., Kirsch, I., Kong, J., Wasan, A. D., & Napadow, V. (2013). Default mode network connectivity encodes clinical pain: An arterial spin labeling study. *Pain*, *154*(1), 24–33.

Louise, S., Fitzpatrick, M., Strauss, C., Rossell, S. L., & Thomas, N. (2018). Mindfulness- and acceptance-based interventions for psychosis: Our current understanding and a meta-analysis. *Schizophrenia Research*, *192*, 57–63.

Lubman, D. I., Allen, N. B., Peters, L. A., & Deakin, J. F. (2008). Electrophysiological evidence that drug cues have greater salience than other affective stimuli in opiate addiction. *Journal of Psychopharmacology*, *22*, 836–842.

Lubman, D. I., Yucel, M., Kettle, J. W., Scaffidi, A., Mackenzie, T., Simmons, J. G., & Allen, N. B. (2009). Responsiveness to drug cues and natural rewards in opiate addiction: Associations with later heroin use. *Archives of General Psychiatry*, *66*, 205–212.

Lundberg, U., Dohns, I. E., Melin, B., Sandsjö, L., Palmerud, G., Kadefors, R., Ekström, M., & Parr, D. (1999). Psychophysiological stress responses, muscle tension, and neck and shoulder pain among supermarket cashiers. *Journal of Occupational Health Psychology*, *4*(3), 245–255.

Lutz, A., Slagter, H. A., Dunne, J. D., & Davidson, R. J. (2008). Attention regulation and monitoring in meditation. *Trends in Cognitive Science*, *12*, 163–169.

Lutz, A., & Thompson, E. (2003). Neurophenomenology integrating subjective experience and brain dynamics in the neuroscience of consciousness. *Journal of Consciousness Studies*, *10*(9–10), 31–52.

Mackey, K., Anderson, J., Bourne, D., Chen, E., & Peterson, K. (2020). Benefits and harms of long-term opioid dose reduction or discontinuation in patients with chronic pain: A rapid review. *Journal of General Internal Medicine*, *35*(3), 935–944.

Marlatt, G. A., & Donovan, D. M. (Eds.). (2005). *Relapse prevention: Maintenance strategies in the treatment of addictive behaviors* (2nd ed.). Guilford Press.

Martel, M. O., Dolman, A. J., Edwards, R. R., Jamison, R. N., & Wasan, A. D. (2014). The association between negative affect and prescription opioid misuse in patients with chronic pain: The mediating role of opioid craving. *Journal of Pain*, *15*(1), 90–100.

Mathieu-Kia, A. M., Fan, L. Q., Kreek, M. J., Simon, E. J., & Hiller, J. M. (2001). Mu-, delta- and kappa-opioid receptor populations are differentially altered in distinct areas of postmortem brains of Alzheimer's disease patients. *Brain Research*, *893*(1), 121–134.

Matt, D. C. (1995). *The essential Kabbalah: The heart of Jewish Mysticism*. HarperCollins.

Maturana, H., & Varela, F. (1987). *The tree of knowledge: The biological roots of human understanding*. Shambhala.

Meier, I. M., Eikemo, M., & Leknes, S. (2021). The role of mu-opioids for reward and threat processing in humans: Bridging the gap from preclinical to clinical opioid drug studies. *Current Addiction Reports*, *8*, 306–318.

Melzack, R., & Wall, P. D. (1965). Pain mechanisms: A new theory. *Science*, *150*(699), 971–979.

Metzinger, T. (2024). *The elephant and the blind: The experience of pure consciousness—Philosophy, science, and 500+ experiential reports*. MIT Press.

Miller, W. R. (1983). Motivational interviewing with problem drinkers. *Behavioural Psychotherapy*, *11*(2), 147–172.

Miller, W. R., & Rollnick, S. (2023). *Motivational interviewing: Helping people change and grow* (4th ed.). Guilford Press.

Moseley, J. B., O'Malley, K., Petersen, N. J., Menke, T. J., Brody, B. A., Kuykendall, D. H., Hollingsworth, J. C., Ashton, C. M., & Wray, N. P. (2002). A controlled trial of arthroscopic surgery for osteoarthritis of the knee. *New England Journal of Medicine, 347*(2), 81–88.

Namgyal, D. T. (2006). *Mahamudra: The moonlight–quintessence of mind and meditation.* Simon & Schuster.

Namgyal, D. T. (2019). *Moonbeams of Mahamudra.* Shambhala.

Nelson, T. O., Stuart, R. B., Howard, C., & Crowley, M. (1999). Metacognition and clinical psychology: A preliminary framework for research and practice. *Clinical Psychology and Psychotherapy, 6*, 73–79.

Norbu, C. N., & Clemente, A. (1999). *The supreme source: The fundamental tantra of Dzogchen Semde Kunjed Gyalpo.* Shambhala.

Nyanaponika. (1998). *Abhidhamma studies: Buddhist explorations of consciousness and time.* Simon & Schuster.

Ochsner, K. N., & Gross, J. J. (2005). The cognitive control of emotion. *Trends in Cognitive Science, 9*(5), 242–249.

Olds, J., & Milner, P. (1954). Positive reinforcement produced by electrical stimulation of septal area and other regions of rat brain. *Journal of Comparative and Physiological Psychology, 47*(6), 419–427.

Pan, Y. X., & Pasternak, G. W. (2011). Molecular biology of mu opioid receptors. *Opiate Receptors*, 121–160.

Panerai, A. E. (2011). Pain emotion and homeostasis. *Neurological Sciences, 32*(S1), 27–29.

Pantazis, C. B., Gonzalez, L. A., Tunstall, B. J., Carmack, S. A., Koob, G. F., & Vendruscolo, L. F. (2021). Cues conditioned to withdrawal and negative reinforcement: Neglected but key motivational elements driving opioid addiction. *Science Advances, 7*(15), eabf0364.

Parisi, A., Roberts, R. L., Hanley, A. W., & Garland, E. L. (2022). Mindfulness-oriented recovery enhancement for addictive behavior, psychiatric distress, and chronic pain: A multilevel meta-analysis of randomized controlled trials. *Mindfulness, 13*(10), 2396–2412.

Petitmengin, C., van Beek, M., Bitbol, M., & Nissou, J.-M. (2017). What is it like to meditate? Methods and issues for a micro-phenomenological description of meditative experience. *Journal of Consciousness Studies, 24*(5–6), 170–198.

Petrenko, A. B., Yamakura, T., Baba, H., & Shimoji, K. (2003). The role of N-methyl-D-aspartate (NMDA) receptors in pain: A review. *Anesthesia and Analgesia, 97*(4), 1108–1116.

Piazza, P. V., & Deroche-Gamonet, V. (2013). A multistep general theory of transition to addiction. *Psychopharmacology, 229*(3), 387–413.

Picavet, H. S. J., Vlaeyen, J. W. S., & Schouten, J. S. A. G. (2002). Pain catastrophizing and kinesiophobia: Predictors of chronic low back pain. *American Journal of Epidemiology, 156*(11), 1028–1034.

Potter, J. S., Chakrabarti, A., Domier, C. P., Hillhouse, M. P., Weiss, R. D., & Ling, W. (2010). Pain and continued opioid use in individuals receiving buprenorphine–naloxone for opioid detoxification: Secondary analyses from the Clinical Trials Network. *Journal of Substance Abuse Treatment, 38*, S80–S86.

Price, D. D. (2002). Central neural mechanisms that interrelate sensory and affective dimensions of pain. *Molecular Interventions, 2*(6), 392–403.

Priddy, S. E., Hanley, A. W., Riquino, M. R., Platt, K. A., Baker, A. K., & Garland, E. L. (2018). Dispositional mindfulness and prescription opioid misuse among chronic pain patients: Craving and attention to positive information as mediating mechanisms. *Drug and Alcohol Dependence, 188*, 86–93.

Quartana, P. J., Buenaver, L. F., Edwards, R. R., Klick, B., Haythornthwaite, J. A., & Smith, M. T. (2010). Pain catastrophizing and salivary cortisol responses to laboratory pain testing in temporomandibular disorder and healthy participants. *Journal of Pain, 11*(2), 186–194.

Quevedo, A. S., & Coghill, R. C. (2007). Attentional modulation of spatial integration of pain: Evidence for dynamic spatial tuning. *Journal of Neuroscience, 27*(43), 11635–11640.

Rahula, W. (2007). *What the Buddha taught.* Grove Press. (Original work published 1959)

Raichle, M. E., MacLeod, A. M., Snyder, A. Z., Powers, W. J., Gusnard, D. A., & Shulman, G. L. (2001). A default mode of brain function. *Proceedings of the National Academy of Sciences, 98*(2), 676–682.

Rainville, P., Bao, Q. V. H., & Chrétien, P. (2005). Pain-related emotions modulate experimental pain perception and autonomic responses. *Pain, 118*(3), 306–318.

Rainville, P., Carrier, B., Hofbauer, R. K., Bushnell,

M. C., & Duncan, G. H. (1999). Dissociation of sensory and affective dimensions of pain using hypnotic modulation. *Pain, 82,* 159–171.

Rainville, P., Duncan, G. H., Price, D. D., Carrier, B., & Bushnell, M. C. (1997). Pain affect encoded in human anterior cingulate but not somatosensory cortex. *Science, 277,* 968–971.

Raja, S. N., Carr, D. B., Cohen, M., Finnerup, N. B., Flor, H., Gibson, S., Keefe, F. J., Mogil, J. S., Ringkamp, M., Sluka, K. A., Song, X.-J., Stevens, B., Sullivan, M. D., Tutelman, P. R., Ushida, T., & Vader, K. (2020). The revised International Association for the Study of Pain definition of pain: Concepts, challenges, and compromises. *Pain, 161*(9), 1976–1982.

Ray, R. A. (2002). *Secret of the vajra world: The tantric Buddhism of Tibet.* Shambhala.

Reynolds, D. V. (1969). Surgery in the rat during electrical analgesia induced by focal brain stimulation. *Science, 164*(3878), 444–445.

Rinpoche, T. U. (2013). *Quintessential Dzogchen: Confusion dawns as wisdom.* Rangjung Yeshe.

Robinson, T. E., & Berridge, K. C. (2000). The psychology and neurobiology of addiction: An incentive-sensitization view. *Addiction, 95*(Suppl. 2), S91–S117.

Rogers, A. H., Zvolensky, M. J., Ditre, J. W., Buckner, J. D., & Asmundson, G. J. (2021). Association of opioid misuse with anxiety and depression: A systematic review of the literature. *Clinical Psychology Review,* 101978.

Rohsenow, D. J., Monti, P. M., Rubonis, A. V., Sirota, A. D., Niaura, R. S., Colby, S. M., Wunschel, S. M., & Abrams, D. B. (1994). Cue reactivity as a predictor of drinking among male alcoholics. *Journal of Consulting and Clinical Psychology, 62*(3), 620.

Rollman, G. B. (2009). Perspectives on hypervigilance. *Pain, 141*(3), 183–184.

Rothberg, R. L., Azhari, N., Haug, N. A., & Dakwar, E. (2021). Mystical-type experiences occasioned by ketamine mediate its impact on at-risk drinking: Results from a randomized, controlled trial. *Journal of Psychopharmacology, 35*(2), 150–158.

Roy, M., Piché, M., Chen, J.-I., Peretz, I., & Rainville, P. (2009). Cerebral and spinal modulation of pain by emotions. *Proceedings of the National Academy of Sciences, 106*(49), 20900–20905.

Rubin, R. (2019). HHS guide for tapering or stopping long-term opioid use. *JAMA, 322*(20), 1947.

Rumi, J. (1995). The guest house. In C. Barks with J. Moyne, A. J. Arberry, & R. Nicholson (Trans.), *The essential Rumi* (p. 109). Harper.

Sala, M., Rochefort, C., Lui, P. P., & Baldwin, A. S. (2020). Trait mindfulness and health behaviours: A meta-analysis. *Health Psychology Review, 14*(3), 345–393.

Santo, T., Campbell, G., Gisev, N., Martino-Burke, D., Wilson, J., Colledge-Frisby, S., Clark, B., Tran, L. T., & Degenhardt, L. (2022). Prevalence of mental disorders among people with opioid use disorder: A systematic review and meta-analysis. *Drug and Alcohol Dependence, 238,* 109551.

Schoth, D. E., Nunes, V. D., & Liossi, C. (2012). Attentional bias towards pain-related information in chronic pain: A meta-analysis of visual-probe investigations. *Clinical Psychology Review, 32*(1), 13–25.

Segal, Z. V., Williams, J. M. G., & Teasdale, J. D. (2002). *Mindfulness-based cognitive therapy for depression.* Guilford Press.

Segal, Z., Williams, M., & Teasdale, J. (2013). *Mindfulness-based cognitive therapy for depression* (2nd ed.). Guilford Press.

Seligman, M. E., Rashid, T., & Parks, A. C. (2006). Positive psychotherapy. *American Psychologist, 61,* 774–788.

Severeijns, R., Vlaeyen, J. W. S., van den Hout, M. A., & Weber, W. E. J. (2001). Pain catastrophizing predicts pain intensity, disability, and psychological distress independent of the level of physical impairment. *Clinical Journal of Pain, 17*(2), 165–172.

Shapiro, S. L., Carlson, L. E., Astin, J. A., & Freedman, B. (2006). Mechanisms of mindfulness. *Journal of Clinical Psychology, 62,* 373–386.

Sharp, P. E. (2014). Meditation-induced bliss viewed as release from conditioned neural (thought) patterns that block reward signals in the brain pleasure center. *Religion, Brain and Behavior, 4*(3), 202–229.

Sherman, S. M., & Guillery, R. (1996). Functional organization of thalamocortical relays. *Journal of Neurophysiology, 76*(3), 1367–1395.

Shiffrin, R. M., & Schneider, W. (1977). Controlled and automatic human information processing: II. Perceptual learning, automatic attending and a general theory. *Psychological Review, 84*(2), 127–190.

Shurman, J., Koob, G. F., & Gutstein, H. B. (2010). Opioids, pain, the brain, and hyperkatifeia: A framework for the rational use of opioids for pain. *Pain Medicine, 11*(7), 1092–1098.

Slade, S. C., Molloy, E., & Keating, J. L. (2009). Stigma experienced by people with nonspecific chronic low back pain: A qualitative study. *Pain Medicine, 10*(1), 143–154.

Sommer, C., & Kress, M. (2004). Recent findings on how proinflammatory cytokines cause pain: Peripheral mechanisms in inflammatory and neuropathic hyperalgesia. *Neuroscience Letters, 361*(1–3), 184–187.

Spagnolo, P. A., Kimes, A., Schwandt, M. L., Shokri-Kojori, E., Thada, S., Phillips, K. A., Diazgranados, N., Preston, K. L., Herscovitch, P., Tomasi, D., Ramchandani, V. A., & Heilig, M. (2019). Striatal dopamine release in response to morphine: A [11C]raclopride positron emission tomography study in healthy men. *Biological Psychiatry, 86*(5), 356–364.

Sprenger, C., Eippert, F., Finsterbusch, J., Bingel, U., Rose, M., & Büchel, C. (2012). Attention modulates spinal cord responses to pain. *Current Biology, 22*(11), 1019–1022.

Stanko, K. E., Cherry, K. E., Ryker, K. S., Mughal, F., Marks, L. D., Brown, J. S., Gendusa, P. F., Sullivan, M. C., Bruner, J., Welsh, D. A., Su, L. J., & Jazwinski, S. M. (2015). Looking for the silver lining: Benefit finding after Hurricanes Katrina and Rita in middle-aged, older, and oldest-old adults. *Current Psychology, 34*(3), 564–575.

Stein, E. M., Gennuso, K. P., Ugboaja, D. C., & Remington, P. L. (2017). The epidemic of despair among White Americans: Trends in the leading causes of premature death, 1999–2015. *American Journal of Public Health, 107*(10), 1541–1547.

Strick, M., van Noorden, T. H., Ritskes, R. R., de Ruiter, J. R., & Dijksterhuis, A. (2012). Zen meditation and access to information in the unconscious. *Consciousness and Cognition, 21*(3), 1476–1481.

Strigo, I. A., Simmons, A. N., Matthews, S. C., Craig, A. D. (Bud), & Paulus, M. P. (2008). Increased affective bias revealed using experimental graded heat stimuli in young depressed adults: Evidence of "emotional allodynia." *Psychosomatic Medicine, 70*(3), 338–344.

Substance Abuse and Mental Health Services Administration (SAMHSA). (2011). *Recovery and recovery support.* www.samhsa.gov/find-help/recovery

Substance Abuse and Mental Health Services Administration (SAMHSA). (2012). *Working definition of recovery.* https://store.samhsa.gov/system/files/pep12-recdef.pdf

Substance Abuse and Mental Health Services Administration (SAMHSA). (2023). *The National Survey on Drug Use and Health (NSDUH): 2022.* www.samhsa.gov/data/release/2022-national-survey-drug-use-and-health-nsduh-releases

Sullivan, M. D., Edlund, M. J., Fan, M. Y., Devries, A., Brennan Braden, J., & Martin, B. C. (2010). Risks for possible and probable opioid misuse among recipients of chronic opioid therapy in commercial and Medicaid insurance plans: The TROUP study. *Pain, 150,* 332–339.

Sumantry, D., & Stewart, K. E. (2021). Meditation, mindfulness, and attention: A meta-analysis. *Mindfulness, 12,* 1332-1349.

Tagliazucchi, E., Roseman, L., Kaelen, M., Orban, C., Muthukumaraswamy, S. D., Murphy, K., Laufs, H., Leech, R., McGonigle, J., Crossley, N., Bullmore, E., Williams, T., Bolstridge, M., Feilding, A., Nutt, D. J., & Carhart-Harris, R. (2016). Increased global functional connectivity correlates with LSD-induced ego dissolution. *Current Biology, 26*(8), 1043–1050.

Tang, R., Friston, K. J., & Tang, Y.-Y. (2020). Brief mindfulness meditation induces gray matter changes in the brain hub. *Neural Plasticity, 2020,* 8830005.

Tang, Y.-Y., Hölzel, B. K., & Posner, M. I. (2015). The neuroscience of mindfulness meditation. *Nature Reviews Neuroscience, 16*(4), 213–225.

Tang, Y.-Y., Lu, Q., Fan, M., Yang, Y., & Posner, M. I. (2012). Mechanisms of white matter changes induced by meditation. *Proceedings of the National Academy of Sciences, 109*(26), 10570–10574.

Tang, Y.-Y., Lu, Q., Geng, X., Stein, E. A., Yang, Y., & Posner, M. I. (2010). Short-term meditation induces white matter changes in the anterior cingulate. *Proceedings of the National Academy of Sciences, 107*(35), 15649–15652.

Teasdale, J. D., Segal, Z. V., Williams, J. M. G., Ridgeway, V. A., Soulsby, J. M., & Lau, M. A. (2000). Prevention of relapse/recurrence in major depression by mindfulness-based cognitive therapy. *Journal of Consulting and Clinical Psychology, 68*(4), 615.

Teasdale, J. (2022). *What happens in mindfulness: Inner awakening and embodied cognition.* Guilford Press.

Terkelsen, A. J., Andersen, O. K., Mølgaard, H., Hansen, J., & Jensen, T. (2004). Mental stress inhibits pain perception and heart rate variability but not a nociceptive withdrawal reflex. *Acta Physiologica Scandinavica, 180*(4), 405–414.

Thomas, E. A., Mijangos, J. L., Hansen, P. A., White, S., Walker, D., Reimers, C., Beck, A. C., & Garland, E. L. (2019). Mindfulness-oriented recovery enhancement restructures reward processing and promotes interoceptive awareness in overweight cancer survivors: Mechanistic results from a stage 1 randomized controlled trial. *Integrative Cancer Therapies, 18,* 1534735419855138.

Tiffany, S. T. (1990). A cognitive model of drug urges and drug-use behavior: Role of automatic and nonautomatic processes. *Psychological Review, 97,* 147–168.

Tolin, D. F. (2010). Is cognitive-behavioral therapy more effective than other therapies? A meta-analytic review. *Clinical Psychology Review, 30,* 710–720.

Tracey, I., & Mantyh, P. W. (2007). The cerebral signature for pain perception and its modulation. *Neuron, 55*(3), 377–391.

Traynor, J. R., & Wood, M. S. (1987). Distribution of opioid binding sites in spinal cord. *Neuropeptides, 10*(4), 313–320.

Trungpa, C. (1985). *Shambhala: The sacred path of the warrior.* Shambhala.

Tsongkhapa, J. (2012). *A lamp to illuminate the five stages: Teachings on Guhyasamaja Tantra* (Vol. 15). Simon & Schuster.

Turk, D. C., & Flor, H. (1987). Pain greater than pain behaviors: The utility and limitations of the pain behavior construct. *Pain, 31*(3), 277–295.

Vago, D. R., & Silbersweig, D. A. (2012). Self-awareness, self-regulation, and self-transcendence (S-ART): A framework for understanding the neurobiological mechanisms of mindfulness. *Frontiers in Human Neuroscience, 6,* 296.

Valet, M., Sprenger, T., Boecker, H., Willoch, F., Rummeny, E., Conrad, B., Erhard, P., & Tolle, T. R. (2004). Distraction modulates connectivity of the cingulo-frontal cortex and the midbrain during pain—an fMRI analysis. *Pain, 109*(3), 399–408.

Valk, S. L., Bernhardt, B. C., Trautwein, F.-M., Böckler, A., Kanske, P., Guizard, N., Collins, D. L., & Singer, T. (2017). Structural plasticity of the social brain: Differential change after socio-affective and cognitive mental training. *Science Advances, 3*(10), e1700489.

Varela, F., Thompson, E., & Rosch, E. (1991). *The embodied mind: Cognitive science and human experience.* MIT Press.

Vest, N. A., McPherson, S., Burns, G. L., & Tragesser, S. (2020). Parallel modeling of pain and depression in prediction of relapse during buprenorphine and naloxone treatment: A finite mixture model. *Drug and Alcohol Dependence, 209,* 107940.

Vieten, C., Wahbeh, H., Cahn, B. R., MacLean, K., Estrada, M., Mills, P., Murphy, M., Shapiro, S., Radin, D., Josipovic, Z., Presti, D. E., Sapiro, M., Bays, J. C., Russell, P., Vago, D., Travis, F., Walsh, R., & Delorme, A. (2018). Future directions in meditation research: Recommendations for expanding the field of contemplative science. *PLOS ONE, 13*(11), e0205740.

Vlaeyen, J. W., & Linton, S. J. (2012). Fear-avoidance model of chronic musculoskeletal pain: 12 years on. *Pain, 153*(6), 1144–1147.

Voisin, D. L., Guy, N., Chalus, M., & Dallel, R. (2005). Nociceptive stimulation activates locus coeruleus neurones projecting to the somatosensory thalamus in the rat. *Journal of Physiology, 566*(3), 929–937.

Volkow, N. D., Michaelides, M., & Baler, R. (2019). The neuroscience of drug reward and addiction. *Physiological Reviews, 99*(4), 2115–2140.

Volkow, N. D., Wang, G.-J., Fowler, J. S., Tomasi, D., & Telang, F. (2011). Addiction: Beyond dopamine reward circuitry. *Proceedings of the National Academy of Sciences, 108*(37), 15037–15042.

Vowles, K. E., McEntee, M. L., Julnes, P. S., Frohe, T., Ney, J. P., & van der Goes, D. N. (2015). Rates of opioid misuse, abuse, and addiction in chronic pain: A systematic review and data synthesis. *Pain, 156*(4), 569–576.

Vygotsky, L. S. (1978). *Mind in society: The development of higher psychological processes.* Harvard University Press.

Wager, T. D., Davidson, M. L., Hughes, B. L., Lindquist, M. A., & Ochsner, K. N. (2008). Prefrontal-subcortical pathways mediating successful emotion regulation. *Neuron, 59*(6), 1037–1050.

Wager, T. D., Scott, D. J., & Zubieta, J.-K. (2007). Placebo effects on human μ-opioid activity during pain. *Proceedings of the National Academy of Sciences, 104*(26), 11056–11061.

Wahbeh, H., Sagher, A., Back, W., Pundhir, P., & Travis, F. (2018). A systematic review of transcendent states across meditation and contemplative traditions. *Explore, 14*(1), 19–35.

Wallis, C. D. (2017). *The recognition sutras: Illuminating a 1,000-year-old spiritual masterpiece.* Mattamayura Press.

Wang, Y., Garland, E. L., & Farb, N. A. (2023). An experimental test of the mindfulness-to-meaning theory: Causal pathways between decentering, reappraisal, and wellbeing. *Emotion, 23*(8), 2243–2258.

Wanigasekera, V., Lee, M. C., Rogers, R., Kong, Y.,

Leknes, S., Andersson, J., & Tracey, I. (2012). Baseline reward circuitry activity and trait reward responsiveness predict expression of opioid analgesia in healthy subjects. *Proceedings of the National Academy of Sciences, 109*(43), 17705–17710.

Wasan, A. D., Loggia, M. L., Chen, L. Q., Napadow, V., Kong, J., & Gollub, R. L. (2011). Neural correlates of chronic low back pain measured by arterial spin labeling. *Anesthesiology, 115*(2), 364–374.

Watts, A. W. (1989). *Psychotherapy east and west.* New World Library. (Original work published 1961)

Watts, A. W. (2011). *The book: On the taboo against knowing who you are.* Vintage. (Original work published 1959)

Wegner, D. M. (1994). Ironic processes of mental control. *Psychological Review, 101*, 34–52.

Wenk-Sormaz, H. (2005). Meditation can reduce habitual responding. *Alternative Therapies in Health and Medicine, 11*, 42–58.

Wiech, K. (2016). Deconstructing the sensation of pain: The influence of cognitive processes on pain perception. *Science, 354*(6312), 584–587.

Wiech, K., Kalisch, R., Weiskopf, N., Pleger, B., Stephan, K. E., & Dolan, R. J. (2006). Anterolateral prefrontal cortex mediates the analgesic effect of expected and perceived control over pain. *Journal of Neuroscience, 26*(44), 11501–11509.

Wiech, K., Ploner, M., & Tracey, I. (2008). Neurocognitive aspects of pain perception. *Trends in Cognitive Sciences, 12*(8), 306–313.

Wiech, K., & Tracey, I. (2009). The influence of negative emotions on pain: Behavioral effects and neural mechanisms. *NeuroImage, 47*(3), 987–994.

Wiers, R. W., Bartholow, B. D., van den Wildenberg, E., Thush, C., Engels, R. C., Sher, K. J., Grenard, J., Ames, S. L., & Stacy, A. W. (2007). Automatic and controlled processes and the development of addictive behaviors in adolescents: A review and a model. *Pharmacology, Biochemistry, and Behavior, 86*, 263–283.

Willis, W., & Westlund, K. (1997). Neuroanatomy of the pain system and of the pathways that modulate pain. *Journal of Clinical Neurophysiology, 14*(1), 2–31.

Woo, C.-W., Schmidt, L., Krishnan, A., Jepma, M., Roy, M., Lindquist, M. A., Atlas, L. Y., & Wager, T. D. (2017). Quantifying cerebral contributions to pain beyond nociception. *Nature Communications, 8*(1), 1–14.

Worley, M. J., Heinzerling, K. G., Shoptaw, S., & Ling, W. (2015). Pain volatility and prescription opioid addiction treatment outcomes in patients with chronic pain. *Experimental and Clinical Psychopharmacology, 23*(6), 428–435.

Wright, J. H., Brown, G. K., Thase, M. E., & Basco, M. R. (2017). *Learning cognitive-behavior therapy: An illustrated guide.* American Psychiatric.

Wu, S. M., Compton, P., Bolus, R., Schieffer, B., Pham, Q., Baria, A., Van Vort, W., Davis, F., Shekelle, P., & Naliboff, B. D. (2006). The Addiction Behaviors Checklist: Validation of a new clinician-based measure of inappropriate opioid use in chronic pain. *Journal of Pain and Symptom Management, 32*(4), 342–351.

Yaden, D. B., Haidt, J., Hood, R. W., Jr., Vago, D. R., & Newberg, A. B. (2017). The varieties of self-transcendent experience. *Review of General Psychology, 21*(2), 143–160.

Yaksh, T. L. (1985). Pharmacology of spinal adrenergic systems which modulate spinal nociceptive processing. *Pharmacology, Biochemistry, and Behavior, 22*(5), 845–858.

Yaksh, T. L. (1987). Opioid receptor systems and the endorphins: A review of their spinal organization. *Journal of Neurosurgery, 67*(2), 157–176.

Yapko, M. D. (2011). *Mindfulness and hypnosis: The power of suggestion to transform experience.* Norton.

Yapko, M. D. (2020). Contemplating . . . the obvious: What you focus on, you amplify. *International Journal of Clinical and Experimental Hypnosis, 68*(2), 144–150.

Yin, H. H., & Knowlton, B. J. (2006). The role of the basal ganglia in habit formation. *Nature Reviews Neuroscience, 7*, 464–476.

Zacny, J. P. (1995). A review of the effects of opioids on psychomotor and cognitive functioning in humans. *Experimental and Clinical Psychopharmacology, 3*(4), 432–466.

Zeidan, F., & Coghill, R. C. (2013). Functional connections between self-referential thought and chronic pain: A dysfunctional relationship. *Pain, 154*(1), 3–4.

Zeidan, F., Emerson, N. M., Farris, S. R., Ray, J. N., Jung, Y., McHaffie, J. G., & Coghill, R. C. (2015). Mindfulness meditation-based pain relief employs different neural mechanisms than placebo and sham mindfulness meditation-induced analgesia. *Journal of Neuroscience, 35*(46), 15307–15325.

Zeidan, F., Martucci, K. T., Kraft, R. A., Gordon, N. S., McHaffie, J. G., & Coghill, R. C. (2011). Brain mechanisms supporting the modulation of pain by mindfulness meditation. *Journal of Neuroscience, 31*(14), 5540–5548.

Zhang, R., & Volkow, N. D. (2019). Brain default-mode network dysfunction in addiction. *NeuroImage, 200*, 313–331.

Index

Note. *f* or *t* following a page number indicates a figure or table.